D0930315

MANAGING INSTITUTIONAL PLANNING

Health Facilities and PL 93-641

Martin S. Perlin, D.B.A.

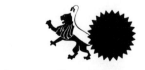

Aspen Systems Corporation
Germantown, Maryland
1976

"This publication is designed to provide accurate and authoritative information in regard to the Subject Matter covered. It is sold with the understanding that the publisher is not engaged in rendering legal, accounting, or other professional service. If legal advice or other expert assistance is required, the services of a competent professional person should be sought." From a Declaration of Principles jointly adopted by a Committee of the American Bar Association and a Committee of Publishers and Associations.

Library of Congress Catalog Card Number: 76-29788
ISBN:0-912862-31-9

Printed in the United States of America

1 2 3 4 5

Dedicated To
Madeleine, Melina, Michael, and Marc

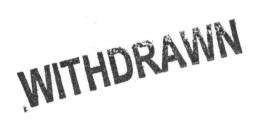

Table of Contents

List of Tables and Figures

List of Abbreviations

ACHA   American College of Hospital Administrators

ACME   Association of Consulting Management Engineers

AIP   Annual Implementation Plan

CHPA   Comprehensive Health Planning Agency

DPA   Designated Planning Agency

HEW   Department of Health, Education, and Welfare

HMO   Health Maintenance Organization

HSA   Health Systems Agency

HSP   Health Systems Plan

PSRO   Professional Standards Review Organization

Preface

Formal planning by health institutions has come of age. At the writing of this book the National Health Planning Resources and Development Act (P.L. 93-641) is being implemented through the establishment of a nationwide network of Health Systems Agencies, and under the law all states will be required to enact Certificate of Need laws by 1980. Hospitals and other health institutions are now expected to establish formal planning mechanisms and utilize planning methods with recognized validity to receive approval for program or facility expansion. Expansion funds through public or private means are being tied to facility plans based on sound and defensible planning processes.

To help administrators respond to these new challenges, this book describes the planning structures, processes, and methods that are being successfully adopted by health institutions. Numerous actual examples are provided to demonstrate both the successes and the failures in institutional planning so one might learn from past experiences in shaping a planning program that meets unique institutional environments.

This book is intended to be a practical text on alternatives to establishing and carrying out formal planning in institutions. The book begins with a description of the specific institutional planning requirements under the Health Planning Resource and Development Act. The remainder of the book focuses on the structure, analysis, and methods of planning with examples of how a variety of health institutions carry out this important top management function. Given the increasing regulation and control over the health institution planning process, this book is written from the perspective of the health institution executive whose responsibility is to guide his institution through a planning process that will meet public expectations and regulations.

Acknowledgements

There are a few people I would like to mention who provided invaluable assistance to me during the development of this book. Dr. Larry Prybil provided an environment which encouraged professional development and allowed sufficient time to pursue research interests and writing. The 1975 graduating class in hospital administration at the Medical College of Virginia heard many of my early ideas about hospital planning, challenged my notions and sharpened my thinking. My lecture notes for them served as a basis for many parts of the text. Mr. Joel May, Mr. Frank Reiner and Mr. Richard Clark each read the entire manuscript and offered a number of constructive criticisms which strengthened the final product.

Chapter 1

Planning Laws and Health Facility Requirements

PLANNING RESPONSIBILITIES OF TOP MANAGEMENT

Long as well as short range planning is the responsibility of the top management of any organization. Although hospital executives for many years have engaged in some form of planning for their organizations it has typically been of short duration or has taken place primarily when facility expansion, modernization, or replacement is contemplated. Formal planning during these times of an institution's growth is certainly necessary, but it is not sufficient to meet top management's planning responsibilities. The nature of these responsibilities and the legal requirements that make this an important management function are the subjects of this chapter.

Planning is universally recognized as one of the prime functions performed by every manager. It was only in the 1960s, however, that a general trend toward developing formal, long range health institution plans became noticeable. Though this trend has been accompanied by wide verbal acceptance in the hospital literature, it has met with far less success and acceptance in practice. Perhaps the most basic barrier to effective development of comprehensive long range planning by health facilities has been the role and duties of the chief executive officer. Historically, hospital chief executives have been users of plans, not planners; primarily responsible and accountable for operating the institution. With little time to formulate plans or play a dominant role in determining broad strategies.

But the role of the chief executive in managing today's health care facility has undergone tremendous transformation. His

1

responsibilities have shifted from a focus on internal operations to a combination of internal operation and external affairs in planning, delivery, and reimbursement. It is estimated that over the past decade the total time of the chief executive directed to external affairs, much of it in planning, has increased from a range of 10 to 25 percent to a range of 25 to 75 percent.[1]

The reasons for these executive role changes spring from the entire spectrum of social changes, and the hospital's expanding role in society. Through a growing array of public expectations and regulatory forces, it is clear that a broadened role of the chief executive must be accepted by both administrative personnel and governing boards if the needs of the health facility and the community are to be effectively met. Such was the conclusion of a special task force created by the American College of Hospital Administrators (ACHA).

What are the management responsibilities implied in the planning or external components of this broadened role of the chief executive? The ACHA Task Force offers a list of duties. In the implementation of these responsibilities the chief executive:

1. establishes an organizational climate in which problems are viewed as challenges and encourages a willingness to undertake difficult assignments;

2. initiates proposals as to what the mission of the hospital should be and what the priority mix and time schedule of programs should be to achieve it;

3. anticipates public expectations for the institution and exercises judgment as to what its response should be, both at present and in the future;

4. initiates proposals on the information system so board members can understand and use the data to control program effectiveness and financial position;

5. initiates proposals for policy changes in response to changing conditions and trends;

6. seeks acceptance of key individuals and groups from both inside and outside the hospital for the approved goals of the institution;

7. plans the course of the organization so it remains financially

and otherwise viable, while responding to public needs and expectations; and

8. provides leadership in orchestrating the human resources inside and outside the organization, including the board members, administrative staff, professional staff, and employees, to develop and execute the organization's mission and programs.[2]

In exercising these responsibilities the chief executive faces new challenges and public expectations. The planning requirements of his role have become formalized through the establishment of the National Health Planning Resources and Development Act.

INSTITUTIONAL PLANNING UNDER P.L. 93-641

There is no alternative to the development of a formal planning process by today's health institutions. The National Health Planning and Resources Development Act passed by the Congress in January 1975 establishes a network of local health systems agencies (HSAs) with responsibility for reviewing and granting approval for applications for federal funds for health programs; assisting states in reviewing the need for proposed institutional health services; reviewing the appropriateness of existing institutional health services; and making recommendations for expansion, modernization, or construction of health facilities.

Unlike their predecessor, the Comprehensive Health Planning Agencies (CHPA) established under P.L. 89-749, HSAs will have planning clout. By 1980 states will not be eligible to receive any Public Health Service funds unless they have certificate of need laws. These laws, already passed by more than half the state legislatures, require health institutions to receive a legal confirmation that a proposal for expansion, renovation, modernization, or major program development is justified in a defined service area.

Health Systems Agencies will be authorized to deny all federal grants, loans, or loan subsidies under the Public Health Service Act when they deem new program expenditures by health institutions to be inconsistent with state or local health facility plans.

Even if an institution is not seeking federal funds, HSAs will periodically review the "continuing appropriateness" of all institutional services. HSAs can recommend, for example, that hospitals consolidate or terminate services for greater efficiency. According to the law, the results of such a review must be made public, which could seriously jeopardize the continuing survival of institutions not conforming to local requirements. Major third party payers will likely refuse to sign contracts with institutions providing services deemed inappropriate by an HSA, and lending institutions might be skeptical of making loan commitments.

To be prepared to respond successfully to this stiff new planning environment, health institutions can implement one of two strategies: (1) become actively involved in the organization and decision-making apparatus of the local HSA and attempt to influence the selection or decisions of its members; and (2) become knowledgeable concerning the criteria by which planning efforts will be measured and build an institutional planning process that is prepared to respond to these criteria.

Health Systems Agencies will be one of four types of planning organizations created to carry out the intent of the planning legislation. Each state will designate a *State Health Planning and Development Agency*, which will also be the Designated State Agency that has agreed to implement Sec. 1122 of the Social Security Act.[3] According to the law these agencies will prepare state plans for facility construction, administer a state certificate-of-need program and review existing institutional health services for appropriateness. Each state agency will be advised by a *Statewide Health Coordinating Council*, which will review and coordinate the plans and recommendations of each HSA in its area and will review and approve or disapprove state plans and state health formula grant applications. A *National Council on Health Planning and Development* will advise the Secretary of Health, Education, and Welfare (HEW) on the implementation of the law and recommend national health care priorities.

Individual health institutions and the associations that represent them can seek active involvement in both the Health Systems Agencies and the Statewide Health Coordinating Councils. This involvement can be sought by either obtaining membership on the decision-making bodies governing the activities of these organizations or attempting to influence those who are selected. The governing body of each local HSA normally will have between ten and thirty members, the majority of whom are health care consumers broadly representative of the social, economic, and racial population of the area. The remainder of the membership must represent the health field, including at least one-third who are direct providers of care, such as physicians or administrators. The law does permit the creation of a larger body, with the selection of an executive committee composed as described above. Each Statewide Health Coordinating Council will have at least 60 percent of its members appointed by the governor from nominations from the membership of local HSAs. Each must have a consumer majority.

Once organized, after having been designated by HEW with the advice of state governors, each HSA will turn to its charge as specified in the law. In general, HSAs will be responsible for carrying out the following:

1. implement plans to improve community health;

2. increase accessibility, acceptability, continuity, and quality of health services;

3. restrain increases in health care costs;

4. prevent unnecessary duplication of health services;

5. develop short and long range community health plans; and

6. determine institutional eligibility for all federal health services development funds.

Underlying the charge of each HSA are national health priorities found in Section 1502 of the planning law. In the future, the goals and accomplishments of health institutions are likely to be measured against these national priorities established by Congress, and HSAs will be expected to develop "Health System Plans (HSP)" for their designated areas that implement these priorities.[4]

Sec. 1502, The Congress finds that the following deserve priority consideration in the formulation of national health planning goals and in the development and operations of Federal, State, and area health planning and resources development programs:

(1) The provision of primary care services for medically underserved populations, especially those

which are located in rural or economically depressed areas.

(2) The development of multi-institutional systems for coordination or consolidation of institutional health services.

(3) The development of medical group practices (especially those whose services are appropriately coordinated or integrated with institutional health services), health maintenance organizations, and other organized systems for the provision of health care.

(4) The training and increased utilization of physician assistants, especially nurse clinicians.

(5) The development of multi-institutional arrangements for the sharing of support services necessary to all health service institutions.

(6) The promotion of activities to achieve needed improvements in the quality of health services, including needs identified by the review activities or Professional Standards Review Organizations under part B of title XI of the Social Security Act.

(7) The development by health service institutions of the capacity to provide various levels of care (including intensive care, acute general care, and extended care) on a geographically integrated basis.

(8) The promotion of activities for the prevention of disease, including studies of nutritional and environment factors affecting health and the provision of preventive health care services.

(9) The adoption of uniform cost accounting, simplified reimbursement, and utilization reporting systems, and improved management procedures for health service institutions.

(10) The development of effective methods of educating the general public conerning proper personal (including preventive) health care and methods for effective use of available health services.

Health Systems Agencies will derive their planning muscle from two separate authorizations. First, each agency will have authority to review and approve or disapprove applications for federal funds to develop new institutional programs or to deny federal reimbursement for services that an HSA deems unneeded in a community. Second, each agency will be authorized the direct expenditure of considerable sums of money to start up, organize, and staff health services they deem necessary.[5] In other words, if existing community health institutions are not interested in developing new or expanded services judged by the HSA to be needed, then seed money will be *available to help* those citizens or community groups that are.

The procedures and criteria that will guide HSA reviews of proposed health systems changes are spelled out in the legislation. While they may vary according to the particular purpose or nature of the review, the general intent of Congress is quite clear. To enforce recognized guidelines for project review uniformly throughout the country.

Sec. 1532. (a) In conducting reviews pursuant to subsections (c), (f), and (g) of section 1513 or in conducting any other reviews of proposed or existing health services, each health systems agency shall (except to the extent approved by the Secretary) follow procedures, and apply criteria, developed and published by the agency in accordance with regulations of the Secretary; and in performing its review functions under section 1523, a State Agency shall (except to the extent approved by the Secretary) follow procedures, and apply criteria, developed and published by the State Agency in accordance with regulations of the Secretary. Procedures and criteria for reviews by health systems agencies and State Agencies may vary according to the purpose for which a particular review is being conducted or the type of health services being reviewed.

(b) Each health systems agency and State Agency shall include in the procedures required by subsection (a) at least the following:

(1) Written notification to affected persons of the beginning of a review.

(2) Schedules for reviews which provide that no review shall, to the extent practicable, take longer than ninety days from the date the notification described in paragraph (1) is made.

(3) Provision for persons subject to a review to submit to the agency or State Agency (in such form and manner as the agency or State Agency shall prescribe and publish) such information as the agency or State Agency may require concerning the subject of such review.

(4) Submission of applications (subject to review by a health systems agency or a State Agency) made under this Act or other provisions of law for Federal financial assistance for health services to the health systems agency or State Agency at such time and in such manner as it may require.

(5) Submission of periodic reports by providers of health services and other persons subject to agency or State Agency review respecting the development of proposals subject to review.

(6) Provision for written findings which state the basis for any final decision or recommendation made by the agency or State Agency.

(7) Notification of providers of health services and other persons subject to agency or State Agency review of the status of the agency or State Agency review of the health services or proposals subject to review, findings made in the course of such review, and other appropriate information respecting such review.

(8) Provision for public hearings in the course of agency or State Agency review if requested by persons directly affected by the review; and provision for public hearings, for good cause shown, respecting agency and State Agency decisions.

(9) Preparation and publication of regular reports by the agency and State Agency of the reviews being conducted (including a statement concerning the status of each such review) and of the reviews completed by the agency and State Agency (including a general state-

ment of the findings and decisions made in the course of such reviews) since the publication of the last such report.

(10) Access by the general public to all applications reviewed by the agency and State Agency and to all other written materials pertinent to any agency or State Agency review.

(11) In the case of construction projects, submission to the agency and State Agency by the entities proposing the projects of letters of intent in such detail as may be necessary to inform the agency and State Agency of the scope and nature of the projects at the earliest possible opportunity in the course of planning of such construction projects.

(c) Criteria required by subsection (a) for health systems agency and State Agency review shall include consideration of at least the following:

(1) The relationship of the health services being reviewed to the applicable HSP and AIP.

(2) The relationship of services reviewed to the long-range development plan (if any) of the person providing or proposing such services.

(3) The need that the population served or to be served by such services has for such services.

(4) The availability of alternative, less costly, or more effective methods of providing such services.

(5) The relationship of services reviewed to the existing health care system of the area in which such services are provided or proposed to be provided.

(6) In the case of health services proposed to be provided, the availability of resources (including health manpower, management personnel, and funds for capital and operating needs) for the provision of such services and the availability of alternative uses of such resources, for the provision of other health services.

(7) The special needs and circumstances of those entities which provide a substantial portion of their ser-

vices or resources, or both, to individuals not residing in the health service areas in which the entities are located or in adjacent health service areas. Such entities may include medical and other health professions, schools, multidisciplinary clinics, specialty centers, and such other entities as the Secretary may by regulation prescribe.

(8) The special needs and circumstances of health maintenance organizations for which assistance may be provided under title XIII.

(9) In the case of a construction project—

(A) the costs and methods of the proposed construction, and

(B) the probable impact of the construction project reviewed on the costs of providing health services by the person proposing such construction project.

CRITERIA BY WHICH INSTITUTIONAL PLANNING WILL BE EVALUATED

Each of the project review criteria appearing in Section 1532, subsection C of P.L. 93-641 will have a marked implication on hospital administration. The criteria, as written, established guidelines to be applied by Health Systems Agencies in their review of proposals for program or facility changes. Health institutions will need to understand the full implications of these criteria and create institutional planning processes that are responsive.

Criteria 1. The relationship of the health services being reviewed to the applicable HSP and AIP. The planning law requires each Health System Agency to prepare a long range Health Systems Plan (HSP) and an Annual Implementation Plan (AIP) for its designated area. The HSP will contain a long range statement of area goals and priorities, developed after a detailed analysis of the area and its health care system. The specific contents of the HSP are detailed in the law as follows:

a detailed statement of goals, (A) describing a healthful environment and health systems in the area which, when developed will assure that quality health services will be available and accessible in a manner which assures continuity of care, at reasonable cost, for all residents of the area; (B) which are responsive to the unique needs and resources of the area, and (C) which take into account and are consistent with the national guidelines for health planning under section 1501 respecting supply, distribution, and organization of health resources and services.

The Annual Implementation Plan (AIP) will be a yearly statement of activity required to carry out the long range plan, against which the progress of a health systems agency can be measured.

The first criteria poses the question of whether proposed plans of an institution conform or are consistent with the overall health plans for the community. Paramount in the application of this criteria will be whether the institution, through its proposal, shows evidence of its awareness, support, and desire to participate in the implementation of community health goals adopted by the Health Systems Agency. Second, the institution will need to demonstrate a recognition of community health system priorities as evidenced by its proposed allocation and utilization of resources.

Each HSP will probably contain a development plan for the composition and distribution of health facilities and proposed measures to overcome any gaps in the local health facilities system. An institution's proposed plans of steps to help eliminate system gaps and improve the distribution systems will further demonstrate conformity with the community plan.

Criteria 2. The relationship of services reviewed to the long range development plan of the person providing or proposing such services. In the evaluation of an institution's proposal for changes in the scope or nature of institutional services, an implied assumption will be that there exists a long range plan of development, of which these changes are an integral part. Such a development plan should delineate the institution's mission and role in the community and the long range objectives adopted by the governing body. Reviewing agencies, therefore, would consider that proposed program changes should be an integral part of an overall development plan and should be consistent with the mission, role, and objectives of the institution.

The proposed program should also take place in a time frame that is consistent with the priority needs of the institution. For example, if the correction of licensure or accreditation violations is a logical first phase program, then preceding this with a proposal for adding a parking garage could receive critical review from an HSA. However, the long range plans of an institution must be subjected to periodic review as both external and internal forces place changing demands on an organization. No plan should be so inflexible as to be unable to adjust to changing circumstances. Institutions will need to review and rephrase their long range plans when changes create the need for program proposals that take an institution in new or unplanned directions. They especially will need to demonstrate that these changes emerged from an orderly planning process, with endorsement by the medical staff and governing body, as well as community support.

Criteria 3.   The need that the population served or to be served by such services has for such services.   Each Health Systems Plan will contain an analysis of the community and the "unique needs and resources of the area." This community plan will identify recent and projected demands and resources and outline a plan to overcome unmet needs or gaps in service.

It would therefore be expected that an institution's proposal contain documented demographic data that conforms with that upon which the community health plan is based, and valid projections, which are consistent with community plan projections. Determination of need data should be presented in sufficient detail to demonstrate their validity, and the formulas used to document need should include but not necessarily be limited to those formulas used in the HSP.

The present state of the art in measuring need and demand for health services has not provided uniformly dependable formulas. A number of methodologies exist, each complicated by a number of outside factors, which affect a population's use of services and which are difficult to quantify. Financial or geographic barriers, the way in which health services are organized, and accessibility variations—all impact resulting utilization levels. In presenting need and demand projections, therefore, health institutions should use several acceptable methodologies and formulate expected ranges rather than single projections. When possible, sources of error and potential error magnitudes should support the analysis. As time passes, new data can either confirm or reject previous forecasts and appropriate adjustments can be made in institutional programs. Health institutions often become so dependent on statistical forecasts, which at best are only rough estimates, that they fail to take timely corrective actions when actual data do not support the forecast. Planning on the basis of need and demand projections should, therefore, be subjected to periodic review and refinement as we learn more about how the future actually unfolds.[6]

Criteria 4. The availability of alternative, less costly, or more effective methods of providing such services. Experience to date with planning for health services has shown aptly that a number of options exist in the provision of the same or similar services, often with significant differences in costs. For example, consider the following options which have been implemented by a number of health institutions:

1. ambulatory care programs as alternatives to inpatient care;
2. outpatient surgery as an alternative to inpatient surgery;
3. preadmission testing as an alternative to an extra day's care for patient testing;
4. use of physician extenders where appropriate as an alternative to physicians;
5. home care as an alternative to extended care; and
6. contract for an already existing service as an alternative to providing your own (i.e., shared laundry).

Proposals submitted by health institutions for review will have to demonstrate that alternative solutions have been considered in sufficient detail to assure that the proposed program represents the best solution. Institutions should show evidence that the program will result in the most efficient use of the allocated resources, given program objectives. They should show consideration of alternative health care delivery systems that could improve operating efficiency or reduce operating cost levels. Plans should capitalize on opportunities to improve institutional efficiency by achieving "economies" through shared or merged services. In short, while program options can't be preselected simply on inherent merits, evidence must be present to demonstrate that the institution weighed the efficacy of different alternatives and can justify its choices.

Criteria 5. The relationship of services reviewed to the existing health care system of the area in which such services are provided or proposed to be provided. In the past, many health care facilities have planned independently; little thought was given to the relationship among individual plans and other institutions making up the area's health care delivery system. Under the review of a Health Systems Agency, each health institution will need to provide evidence that its present or proposed program of service is not duplicative of those existing in the community, unless, of course, it can be shown that such duplication is necessary. Further, an estimate should be made of the impact that a proposed program will have on other health care facility utilization in the community, particularly those facilities with common or overlapping service areas.

Institutional plans will have to demonstrate an awareness of an institution's role in the overall community health facility delivery system and a willingness to help correct deficiencies, if they exist, in the distribution of institutional services. In consideration of its community role and long range objectives, an institution will need to take cognizance of how it can participate in the delivery of comprehensive health care services by direct delivery or through effective links with other community agencies or institutions.

Criteria 6. In the case of health services proposed to be provided, the availability of resources (including health manpower, management personnel, and funds for capital and operating needs) for the provision of such services and the availability of alternative uses of such resources for the provision of other health services. Health institutional programs require precious resources, which are scarce in most communities. Health Systems Agencies will have as one of their responsibilities the encouragement of cost-effective use of available resources.

First, an institution will have to provide evidence that sufficient resources can be made available to implement and operate a new program effectively. Putting a new program in place must be followed by operational plans, including life cycle costs, which detail the level of resources required to maintain the program's future viability. But where will the resources come from? What impact, if any, will the proposed program have on manpower distribution and use within the community? Has the institution explored the possibilities of pooling resources through shared services, mergers, or cooperative planning?

Second, in demonstrating the adequacy of monetary resources most institutions will need to have a financial feasibility study conducted. Such a study examines the ability of the institution to borrow or acquire sufficient funds and the capability to pay back debt from future income. If the proposed program is based on a projected demand for service from which future income will be generated, then an examination of the assumptions underlying these projections will be necessary.

Criteria 7.   The special needs and circumstances of those entities that provide a substantial portion of their services or resources, or both, to individuals not residing in the health services areas. Such entities may include medical and other health professions schools, multidisciplinary clinics, specialty centers, and such other entities that the HEW Secretary may by regulation prescribe. Health Systems Agencies will by nature of their local designations and charge, focus their planning and regulatory functions on the unique needs of the populations served in assigned geographic areas. The review and funding mechanisms in the law imply that institutional planning and program proposals will be evaluated against the needs and demands of local communities.

But a number of institutions will provide health services to population groups outside of HSA-designated boundaries. This factor is particularly present in the case of medical centers with large referral caseloads, or multispecialty clinics whose referrals originate on a national or international basis. To address the planning needs of these institutions, the law provides that they be given special consideration in the development of services that are targeted for these special population groups. However, some of these institutions provide a substantial portion of their services to local populations and will, therefore, be subject to HSA review of community need and demand for the services rendered to these groups. A number of referral centers have found that local communities consider these centers as their primary source of care and therefore expect sufficient attention to their needs. Often, the needs of these communities are for a range of primary care services that are not available anywhere else and yet are not of major interest to the institution. While these situations will have to be resolved on a case by case basis, it should be clear that health institutions will be expected to respond to their local neighborhoods if they want continuing community support.

Criteria 8.   The special needs and circumstances of health maintenance organizations for which assistance may be provided under title XIII.   By including special reference to health maintenance organizations (HMOs) in the review criteria, the intent of Congress to give continuing support to the development of these programs is clear. Through the Health Maintenance Organization Act grant money will continue to flow for the planning, organization, and operation of HMOs under a variety of sponsorships. If HSAs are expected to consider the special needs and circumstances of these alternative delivery forms the competitive edge of HMOs in local communities certainly will be sharpened.

.

Criteria 9.   In the case of a construction project, (A) the cost and methods of the proposed construction and (B) the probable impact of the construction project, reviewed on the costs of providing health services by the person proposing such construction project.   Perhaps the major stimulus behind the passage of the National Health Planning and Resources Development Act was the intent to control increases in the cost of health care. In addition to focusing on less costly alternative delivery forms and regulating entry, emphasis would be placed on ways to contain the costs of needed hospital construction. Experience to date has shown that construction costs can be contained through the application of criteria for space allocation; improved methods of design around operational efficiency; the overlapping of design and construction phases; negotiated bidding; the use of standardized components and subassemblies in construction; and the separation in different buildings of services with unlike structural requirements or different growth rates. By one estimate, had these cost containment methods been employed in the construction of all hospitals between 1964 and 1974 savings over traditional methods would have been 30 to 40 percent.[7]

Health institutions contemplating new construction projects will, therefore, have to provide evidence that recognized cost containment methods will be applied whenever feasible, in those cases where new construction is deemed the least costly alternative to the provision of additional services. They will also have to demonstrate that the projected impact of proposed capital expenditures on operating costs will remain within acceptable limits.

Health Systems Agencies should be particularly concerned with the financial impact of capital expenditures on the fiscal structure of an institution. Projections of fiscal performance known as "pro forma" statements should demonstrate a clear prediction of the projects liquidity, including its early years of operation. Further analysis should determine if operating cost levels of a new program and their reflection in patient charges will remain competitive with similar programs in the community.

In the submission of construction project proposals requesting federal financial assistance, health institutions will come under review as specified in Section 1604 of the planning law.

> Sec. 1604. (a) For each project described in section 1601 and included within a State's State medical facilities plan approved under section 1603 there shall be submitted to the Secretary, through the State's State Agency, an application. An application for a grant under section 1625 shall be submitted directly to the Secretary. Except as provided in section 1625, the applicant under such an application may be a State, a political subdivision of a State or any other public entity, or a private non-profit entity. If two or more entities join in a project an application for such project may be filed by any of such entities or by all of them.
> (b) (1) Except as authorized under paragraph (2), an application for any project shall set forth —

(A) in the case of a modernization project for a medical facility for continuation of existing health services, a finding by the State Agency of a continued need for such services, and, in the case of any other project for a medical facility, a finding by the State Agency of the need for the new health services to be provided through the medical facility upon completion of the project;

(B) a description of the site of such project;

(C) plans and specifications therefore which meet the requirements of the regulations prescribed under section 1602(a);

(D) reasonable assurance that title to such site is or will be vested in one or more of the entities filing the application or in a public or other non-profit entity which is to operate the facility on completion of the project;

(E) reasonable assurance that adequate financial support will be available for the completion of the project and for its maintenance and operation when completed, and, for the purpose of determining if the requirements of this subparagraph are met. Federal assistance provided directly to a medical facility which is located in an area determined by the Secretary to be an urban or rural poverty area or through benefits provided individuals served at such facility shall be considered as financial support;

(F) the type of assistance being sought under this title for the project;

(G) except in the case of a project under section 1625, a certification by the State Agency of the Federal share for the project;

(H) reasonable assurance that all laborers and mechanics employed by contractors or subcontractors in the performance of work on a project will be paid wages at rates not less than those prevailing on similar construction in the locality as determined by the Secretary of Labor in accordance with the Act of March 3, 1931 (40 U.S.C. 276a-5, known as the Davis-Bacon Act), and the Secretary of Labor shall have with respect to such labor standards the authority and functions set forth in Reorganization Plan Numbered 14 of 1950 (15 F.R. 3176: 5 U.S.C. Appendix) and section 2 of the Act of June 13, 1934 (40 U.S.C. 276c).

SUMMARY

There is no longer an alternative to formal long range planning by health institutions. The National Health Planning Resources and Development Act (P.L. 93-641), following on the heels of an increasing number of state laws on certificate of need, has set in place a new era in health facility planning. In addition to outside regulations and controls over the operation of health facilities, the top management of today's hospitals must demonstrate that plans for new facilities and major programs are based on sound and defensible planning processes. Those agencies responsible for implementing these regulations will have the necessary clout to make them stick.

Paradoxically, planning has always been a key function of health institution management. But, typically, much planning in the past was in response to critical space needs, utilization problems, or other pressures that can threaten an institution's survival. Historically, health care managers have been users of plans, not planners. Their effort in responding to immediate problems was one of "putting out fires;" and in many cases, the time required for creative future planning was usurped.

However, two major changes in the health industry occurring alongside each other are changing the environment for planning. First, the role of the chief executive is changing its orientation from internal to external. The total time devoted to external affairs is increasing as are the pressures for public accountability and community involvement. This changing orientation of the chief executive is therefore providing a more responsive environment in which regulated planning can flourish. Second, requirements embodied in the new planning law are providing the incentive for institutional planning, which the health industry has not been able to develop voluntarily.

The planning requirements to which the top management of a health institution will have to respond are clear; and, if the intent of the legislation is carried out, these requirements will be administered uniformly throughout the country. The basic criteria by which most institutional planning will be measured can be reduced to seven questions:

1. Does the intent of an institution's plan conform with the goals and objectives of the community's Health System Plan?

2. Does the institution have a long range plan of development of which the proposed project plan is a component part?

3. Can the institution justify a need for the proposed project by the population to be served?

4. Is the proposed project the least costly, most effective alternative for meeting a population need?

5. How will the resources to be devoted to this project relate to and impact on the other health resources in the community?

6. Are the required resources available, and are they the best alternative choice of resources in providing the proposed service?

7. Has the institution considered every available means to achieve cost containment in construction and operation of the proposed project?

In answering the above questions about their planning, health institutions will have to establish formal planning mechanisms and use methods with recognized validity. The following chapters detail this process.

Notes

1. ACHA Task Force V, *Principles of Appointment and Tenure of Executive Officers* (Chicago, Ill.: American College of Hospital Administrators, 1973), p. 3.

2. Ibid., p. 5.

3. Section 221 of P.L. 92-603 created Section 1122 of the Social Security Act. The review and comment process mandated in the legislation to limit federal participation for capital expenditures is under the authority of the State Designated Planning Agencies (DPA).

4. As specified in the legislation, national health priorities will be reviewed and developed further as appropriate, upon recommendation of the National Council on Health Planning and Development.

5. The obligational authority under P.L. 93-641 for development grants for area health

services development funds was $25 million for fiscal year 1975, $75 million for 1976, and $120 million for 1977.

6. For a more detailed discussion of the hazards of predicting the future, see Chapter 4.
7. Hospital Survey Committee, *Cost Containment and Financing of Hospital Construction* (Philadelphia, Pa.: Hospital Survey Committee, 1974), pp. 9-15.

Suggested References

Havighurst, Clark C. *Regulating Health Facilities Construction.* Washington, D.C.: American Enterprise Institute for Public Policy Research, 1974.

Libman, E.W. "Changing Requirements for Approval of Hospital Construction." *Trustee* 25 (Oct. 1972): 20-26.

Reference Manual for Project Review Standards and Criteria. New Orleans: Tulane University, School of Public Health and Tropical Medicine, 1974.

Chapter 2

Creating an Organizational
Climate for Planning

A comprehensive planning program requires a commitment to institutional self-examination, a considerable investment of top management's time, and a willingness to question old ways and adapt to change. Without the proper organizational climate for planning, these requirements are not achievable, and their absence can thwart the entire planning process. The first recommended condition is that the Board of Trustees (or governing body) should be committed to the need to formalize planning.

COMMITMENT OF THE GOVERNING BODY

The overall responsibility for the survival and future of a health institution rests with its governing body. Their past decisions, commitments, and actions, have shaped the organization's nature. A formal planning process challenges these commitments and questions their future applicability, possibly pointing to suggested changes in philosophy or opening up considerations of major changes in institutional goals or programs. Such changes might suggest disbanning old comfortable patterns and moving ahead into unfamiliar waters if the institution is to meet its community and organizational responsibilities. Lacking this understanding and commitment to accept the consequences of the process, little can be accomplished and considerable time and effort can be lost.

Therefore, the governing body must be convinced of the need for and benefits that can be derived from a formal planning process. Most governing bodies have accepted the importance of planning, but in the health field that planning has been chiefly "reactive:"

responding to events, pressures, or crisis. An example of reactive planning is the expansion of a hospital service because of space pressures and/or the political clout of a service director. Although such an expansion might be necessary, it should be part of an overall master plan for facility development and should be weighed against the other competing pressures on an institution. A rational, long range planning approach, in contrast, enables an organization to adapt more readily to future conditions and help shape its own future, to achieve a clear sense of the direction in which it wants to move, and to choose actions that will enable it to accomplish its goals.

Some governing bodies need little convincing that a rational long range planning approach is necessary for the future survival of their health institution. They have witnessed the unending pressures for space and growth and the resulting creation of a maze of poorly integrated facilities in which it is impossible to operate with peak efficiency. They have seen societal, community, and technological pressures for a rate of change in facilities and services against which "reactive" planning has been unable to cope effectively.

As a case in point, take a 450-bed community hospital in a large northeastern city. Pressures for growth had resulted in three separate bed expansions, between 1955 and 1970 bringing the institution from 150 beds to its present complement. With no long range land acquisition program, the location of the new facilities was constrained by a site that became increasingly smaller and more congested with each expansion. During the first two expansions, the pressure for beds and the community appeal of new bed towers had taken priority over ancillary services, which by 1965 were only 50 percent of the size recommended to handle the then existing patient load. The 1965 expansion saw a recognition of this problem, and the Board of Trustees was particularily influenced by a new director of radiology, who demanded a doubling of his department. Site constraints and lack of a previously developed master plan again resulted in a poor solution. The radiology department was doubled in space, however, budget limitations necessitated splitting the department into two locations separated by a long corridor. The resulting impact on operational efficiency should be obvious. By 1970 the hospital site looked like a rat maze, and probably was, for the patient, visitor, and staff, with long horizontal corridors, inadequate elevator service, and an extremely congested hospital site.

Someone had to convince this board of the need for a formal, continuous planning process. An independent evaluation of present facilities, including their operating efficiency and capacity to respond to future needs, might have been a good place to begin. Some institutions have invited outside experts to speak to the governing body on the problems of planning in today's health institutions and the planning requirements and opportunities under federal and state laws. Others have found that private discussions between the chief executive and individual board members about long range planning and the implications for the institution is the preferred approach. But whatever methods are used to convince the board, the implications of their commitment should be clear. Rational long range planning requires time, dedication, and investment. The results of the process can often be painful or, at the least, will question some strongly held notions. Self-assessment is never easy; but to be meaningful, it requires objectivity and commitment to improvement.

FORMALIZING BOARD COMMITMENT

Once an organization agrees to a formally organized planning process, most institutions create a standing committee of the board specifically organized for planning. The committee has been called the long range planning committee, the planning committee, or the planning policy committee. The name is not as important as the committee's composition and charge.

The "planning committee" formalizes the commitment of the governing body to rational planning. As such, its membership should include influential members of the board who are interested in taking part in the manifestation of that commitment and will be able to devote the required time and energy to the planning process.

Commitment to rational planning is also demonstrated by providing on the committee for maximum participation of interested and affected parties. However, the number of committee participants should be held to a manageable size, with the key need being that of providing for a balance of views and perspectives. Each institution will need to determine the composition of the committee in accordance with its own patterns of operation and resources. At a minimum, however most agree that both the administrative and medical staffs of the institution should be represented. Section 234 of P.L. 92-603 states that planning must be under the direction of the governing body by a committee of representatives of that governing body, as well as the administrative and the medical staff of the institution. In most institutions good arguments could be made for including representation from nursing, personnel, finance, and the auxiliary.[1]

While maximum involvement is recommended, most institutions will find it difficult to gain consensus and resolution with a planning committee that has more than six to twelve members. One institution addressed this dilemma by creating a number of subcommittees as part of the parent "planning committee." Subcommittees were created for manpower planning, financial planning, facility planning, and community relations. To give structure and continuity to the process, the planning committee was composed of nine members, including the chairman of each of the subcommittees (see Figure 2.1).

Figure 2.1

**CASE STUDY: ORGANIZATION OF A BOARD PLANNING COMMITTEE
USING SUBCOMMITTEES**

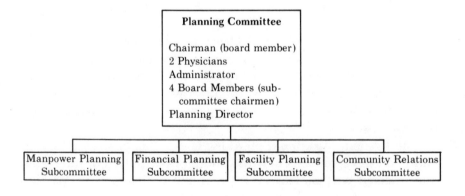

A common mistake is to assign the planning function to the building committee. Although this committee has a crucial role during the planning, design, and construction of a new facility, its focus is usually not broad enough to encompass the full range of planning issues confronting an institution. Building committees are appropriately concerned with bricks and mortar; planning committees are concerned with goals, priorities, options, and institutional strategies. Some institutions might want to consider joint representation between these two committees, as at times their roles are complementary.

THE CHIEF EXECUTIVE'S ROLE

The development of an effective planning program will not be possible in any health institution where the chief executive does not impart firm personal support and commitment throughout the organization. In the absence of his participation and guidance planning will fail. At all levels of organization and management, it should be known that sound planning is considered essential to the health of the institution. The chief executive should ensure that all his managers understand that planning is a continuous function, not one pursued on a one-time basis or only during the annual budgeting process.

One way to demonstrate commitment to the planning process is to create mechanisms to assure meaningful involvement by key decision makers in the organization. With their involvement expected and planning responsibilities delineated, formal planning will be treated much more seriously by more members of the organization. Built into these organizational expectations should be a reward system, which encourages contribution to a sound planning process. One of the major barriers to effective planning by health institutions has been the major emphasis on short term operating results, with the resulting sacrifice of longer range planning results.

One case in point is a 350-bed short term general community hospital in a distant suburb of a major city in the southwest. For many years the hospital had enjoyed the position of being the only hospital in an area for about 150,000 people. To go to alternative facilities, required at least a forty-five minute drive into the city.

This hospitals' occupancy consistently ran over 90 percent even though its facilities were becoming outmoded and were deteriorating in a number of areas. Built in the early 1950s, the hospital had not initiated any major improvements in its facilities since that time, nor had it considered if any changes in role or programs would be required in its long term future. With its high utilization and minimum debt requirements the administrator was able to consistently produce a black bottom line and was rewarded for his ability to maintain hospital facilities at peak utilization. Primarily concerned with the hospital's day-to-day operations, the administrator and his board really had little incentive to look beyond the present year's operating results. While hospital services were not expanding to meet changing community needs, the population and physicians had limited options and, therefore, continued to patronize the institution.

Based on his success in keeping the hospital financially sound, the administrator had many years of employment at this institution. He then accepted a better paying more responsible position only to leave his successor with an outmoded facility that could not meet the changing needs of its community and medical staff. While the former administrator was not measured by his long range planning, the lack of this effort was nearly destructive for the institution.

A number of the hospital's dissatisfied and disgruntled physicians obtained the financial backing of a proprietary hospital chain for the purchase of property (ten miles way from the hospital) on which to construct a new 200-bed hospital.

The group of physicians was able to obtain a certificate of need for the project by carefully demonstrating that it would provide access to a full range of hospital services and that an expanding population could not be adequately accommodated by existing facilities. Missing, for example, were the following services: short term psychiatry, rehabilitation, occupational therapy, and a full range of ambulatory care services. The existing older institution had virtually no training programs for allied health workers which, in part, was responsible for the area's difficulty in employing this needed manpower. Further, it was shown that over the past five years an increasing number of residents were driving considerable distances to other facilities to obtain services not presently provided.

Six months after the new hospital was built, occupancy at the older facility had dropped to 75 percent. Many good physicians switched their institutional loyalties, and the hospital's reputation and survival in the community was a serious question facing its Board of Trustees. Long range planning was initiated through a consultants' study of the situation and the alternatives, but the initiative had been lost. At the present time the newer hospital is considering expansion from 200 to 300 beds on a much sounder base of programs and on well planned structures that can accommodate the expansion. Long range planning and development by the older institution will be an uphill battle all the way.

Long range planning is a difficult job, and there are few tangible measures that can gauge its effectiveness in the short run. There is, naturally, more motivation on the part of operating managers and department heads to spend time on short range planning problems, where measures of performance are more concrete. Lack of effective long range planning often does not show up until the responsible individual has left the institution.

The chief executive, therefore, has to demonstrate by example and actions the importance he places on the planning process. If he devotes time to the process, lower level managers will follow his lead. If he assures that an organization for planning is created with competent guidance and clearly understood procedures, the effort will be taken seriously. If he creates an environment conductive to creative and innovative thinking and the acceptance of change, many individuals participating in that process will receive considerable rewards from the experience.

DEVELOPING ATTITUDES AND PERSPECTIVES

Planning might be necessitated by external pressures to deal with accelerating change or by laws that require a demonstration of planning effort. But *plans* are carried out by people. There are always forces within an organization that operate against a ready reponse to the need for change, and those attitudes can seriously thwart the planning process.

At the top management level and among the leaders of the medical staff some older members with well-established ways of thinking and patterns of doing business could be resistive to initiating change. Others who have benefited from existing programs might have a certain reluctance to change what has worked out well for them. Below the top management level, identifications often are more strongly felt with a functional department than with the organization as a whole, for example, nursing service, food service, radiology, or cardiac surgery. Change, although good for the organization, might weaken or destroy the functional area or might threaten to disturb carefully worked out role and status relationships. Change can also eliminate systems or technologies employees have established or around which they have developed specialized skills or work patterns.

With these organizational "givens" in mind, a planning process, to be effective, must create a climate that will develop the attitudes, perspectives, and personal commitments to make the implementation of plans feasible. Then as circumstances and pressures develop necessitating new changes, these same attitudes, perspectives, and commitments will make continuous planning possible. Flexible and adaptable health institutions are ready to quickly respond to new opportunities, rather than painfully react to building pressures.

But planning often evokes a number of illogical, irrational, and emotional responses, which can seriously inhibit the planning process. According to one management psychologist team, these sometimes unconscious emotional conflicts arise from a dislike of authority, the fear of uncertainty, the fear of failure, and a conflict of indecisiveness.[2] The authority conflict, with its origins in the child's maturation process, forces some adults to rebel against planning if it is perceived as an imposing, directed, or ordered life. Their reaction can be either not to pay attention to plans or to fail to respond properly to plans. The fear of uncertainty conflict arises when lack of information about the future or its effect on an individual's life creates anxiety about losing control over one's own destiny. The result can be an avoidance of planning, pretending that there is no uncertainty and thus formulating unrealistic plans, or setting up a self-fulfilling prophecy by establishing minimal goals with mediocre outcomes. Fear of failure in planning manifests itself in attempts either to avoid planning or to find scapegoats for the errors or stupidity that an individual would choose to avoid at all costs. Finally, the indecisiveness conflict arises out of a desire to avoid self-appraisal and a reexamination of one's goals and direction. Planning can frequently challenge our previous decisions and commitments and make an institution's plans seem indecisive.

It is understandable, then, that those desiring to initiate change in an organization must often cope with both overt and covert resistance to that change, from the top of the organization to the bottom. However, behavioral scientists have been studying the conditions that facilitate the initiation of change and have found that it is possible for management to modify or remove group resistance to change. What is required, they say, is for management to communicate effectively the need for change and to stimulate group participation in planning the changes.[3] Participation by all affected groups helps to establish a shared feeling of need for change, helps to allay misgivings about pending changes, and even can cause a group itself to exert pressures for change.

There are, however, some situations when complete participation by all affected groups has its limitations. One such limitation is when parts of a plan are not to be known by anyone except authorized personnel. Keeping information confidential can give management greater flexibility in some cases, avoid serious embarrassment for the organization, and stop the premature disclosure of a plan before the organization is ready to make an official announcement. A second factor limiting complete participation is the fact that planning often involves behind the scenes maneuvering and a number of strategies designed to channel the planning process. Finally, there is a point at which the advantages of widespread participation in the planning process are outweighed by the disadvantages of cost, delay, and administrative complications of a management system that is too elaborate.

It is the function of management, however, to make proposed changes acceptable to people who are affected by them, if at all possible. Ralph Besse, one highly successful chief executive, has set forth ten guides growing from his experience.

Change is more acceptable when it is understood than when it is not.

Change is more acceptable when it does not threaten security than when it does.

Change is more acceptable when those affected have helped to create it than when it has been externally imposed.

Change is more acceptable when it results from an application of previously established impersonal principles than it is when it is dictated by personal order.

Change is more acceptable when it follows a series of successful changes than it is when it follows a series of failures.

Change is more acceptable when it is inaugurated after prior change has been assimilated than when it is inaugurated during the confusion of other major change.

Change is more acceptable if it has been planned than it is if it is experimental.

Change is more acceptable to people new on the job than to people old on the job.

Change is more acceptable to people who share in the benefits of change than to those who do not.

Change is more acceptable if the organization has been trained to plan for improvement than it is if the organization is accustomed to static procedures.[4]

How does the chief executive evolve a creative and flexible planning climate that builds constructive attitudes and perspectives? One administrator of a 250-bed midwest hospital approached this process cautiously and deliberately. Through numerous one-on-one conversations he tried to establish a mutual understanding of the need for planning and the opportunities that would exist for individuals to become personally involved and have influence over the future plans of the institution. He sought to assure that each individual understood his part in the planning process and accepted it as being important in carrying out his responsibilities in the organization. Finally, in organizing the process he made every attempt to stimulate the flow of ideas, reduce communication blockages, and permit the survival of potentially useful suggestions.

How one achieves these ends in an organization will greatly depend on that organization's history, personnel characteristics, and management style. The process will take the time and patience of all concerned, but the payoff can be dramatic.

START WITH PLANNING SUCCESSES

Once a formal planning process is started it should not be allowed to fail. It might take years to reestablish an organizational climate favorable for another attempt. Therefore, it might be wise to start by solving some simple planning problems before charging into the more complex issues. This gives the board and other participants in the process an opportunity to demonstrate to themselves and others that planning can work. It also gives the planning participants the chance to relate to each other and succeed in that relationship. This success should help to build a foundation of trust and confidence, which will be essential when more difficult and controversial issues are addressed.

An example of how this process worked was observed in a 200-bed hospital in a middle-sized city in Texas. A long range planning committee of the board was appointed to address some critical short term and long term issues facing the institution. Confronted with a changing population composition the institution's historical role as a community hospital serving the needs of a young middle class population was in serious question. Outward migration to the suburbs was resulting in service to a population that was getting increasingly older and less economically well off. There were major differences of opinion among the board and medical staff on what actions should be taken in the long term. Many felt that certain facility limitations were severely constraining the institution from properly responding to immediate needs. For example, the operating suite was considered inadequate in size; there were not enough rooms to accommodate the surgical staff and their patients. There was a proposal to expand the suite immediately by converting adjacent space used for another function and by moving that function to another location. However, the long term implications of this action were instantly recognized. For example, what other areas of the hospital would need to be expanded, and what were the priorities? Was the present location of the operating room suite appropriate for the long term, or would a comprehensive site development plan suggest a different location? One idea emerged from the discussion, however, that offered an immediate solution to improving the situation with a minimum of expense. An outpatient surgery program might relieve some of the pressure on the use of existing operating rooms.

The planning committee, therefore, began its work with examining whether an outpatient surgery program should be instituted. Data was collected supporting the contention that a large percentage of surgical procedures could have been done on an outpatient basis. The literature was reviewed to educate the committee as to the present state of the art. The Director of Finance was asked to provide a report on the financial implications of such a move, and a number of surgeons were asked to express their views. The committee concluded and recommended to the board's Executive Committee that a small outpatient surgical unit be implemented on a trial basis, with an evaluation of the project to be brought back to the committee at the end of six months. The board accepted the recommendations, and the trial unit was established. Encouraged by their success, the planning committee was ready to tackle much more difficult issues.

DEVELOP PLANNING COMPETENCE

The success of the planning effort will, in large measure, depend upon the competence with which planning is carried out. Committees alone will not assure an organized planning approach. Planning committees require competent individuals to staff and guide their activities. Issues must be focused clearly; planning information must be timely, reliable and valid; the costs and benefits of alternative actions should be delineated; and the right people should be involved in the process.

Line management might not have the inclination or temperment and usually will not have the time to devote to the responsibility of organizing and maintaining a long range planning process. Managers who are primarily concerned with acting decisively on short range problems and who have never attempted to formulate broad long range plans and institutional strategies not only will feel uncomfortable but also will lack the preparation and temperment required for the management of the planning effort.

It is, therefore, a major responsibility of the chief executive to assure that a competent planning system is developed and that qualified individuals are selected to guide the process. As the institution's ability and expertise in planning becomes increasingly visible, individuals within the organization are more likely to place confidence in the process and what it can accomplish.

SUMMARY

For a long range planning program to succeed in developing the support and consensus needed for implementation, an organizational climate for planning should be created. Lack of this climate could thwart or otherwise limit the effectiveness of the entire planning process.

The first step is to convince the governing body of the need for a formal, continuing planning process. Then, formalize their commitment through the creation of a top level planning committee with the charge to implement the process. Provide on this committee for the participation of interested and affected parties from both inside and outside the institution, trying to keep the group to a manageable size. Get other members of the institution's management caught up in the "planning fever" by demonstrating that the chief executive takes the process seriously and expects the involvement and creative energies of the entire management team. Build constructive attitudes and perspectives about planning through involvement, discussion, education, and the removal of communication blockages. Without the positive attitudes that this effort can be expected to achieve, overt and covert resistance to change could seriously inhibit the planning process.

Demonstrate that planning can work by using the process and its participants to solve some simple planning problems. Utilize this positive experience to build an environment of trust and confidence, which will be essential for future planning. Carry out the work of planning competently, making sure that qualified individuals are given sufficient time and resources to make planning work. This is the subject of the following chapter.

Notes

1. For an excellent article on establishing a planning committee see J.B. Webber and M.A. Dula, "Effective Planning Committees for Hospitals," *Harvard Business Review* 52, no. 3 (May-June 1974), pp. 133-142.
2. W. Reichman and M. Levy, "Psychological Restraints on Effective Planning," *Management Review* 64, no. 10 (October 1975), pp. 37-42.
3. For several works which support the hypothesis that participation enhances the successful carrying out of planned change see Victor H. Vroom, *Some Personality Determinants of the Effects of Participation* (Englewood Cliffs, N.J.: Prentice-Hall, Inc., 1960); Lester Coch and John R.P. French, Jr., "Overcoming Resistance to Change," in Costello and Zalkind, "Psychology, in Change," *Managing Major Change in Organizations* (Ann Arbor, Michigan: The Foundation for Research on Human Behavior, 1961), pp. 79-81; and H. O. Ronken and Paul R. Lawrence, *Administering Changes* (Boston: Harvard Business School, Division of Research, 1952).
4. Ralph Besse, "Company Planning Must Be Planned," *Dun's Review and Modern Industry* 69, no. 4 (April 1957), pp. 62-63.

Suggested References

Besse, Ralph. "Company Planning Must Be Planned." *Dun's Review and Modern Industry* 69, no. 4 (April 1957): 62-63.

Cummings, Larry. "Organizational Climate for Creativity." *Journal of the Academy of Management* 8, no. 3 (Sept. 1965): 220-227.

Harrison, Roger. "Understanding Your Organization's Character." *Harvard Business Review* 50, no. 3 (May-June 1972): 119-128.

Lawrence, Paul R. "How to Deal with Resistance to Change." *Harvard Business Review* 47, no. 1 (Jan.-Feb. 1969): 4-12, 166-176.

Mann, F.C. and Neff, F.W. "Involvement and Participation in Change." *Managing Major Change in Organizations*. Ann Arbor, Michigan: The Foundation for Research on Human Behavior, 1961: 79-81.

Peters, Joseph P. *Concept Commitment Actions*. New York: United Hospital Fund and the Health and Hospital Planning Council of Southern New York, Inc., 1974. (Also a good reference for Chapters 3, 4, 5, and 6.)

Prince, George M. "Creative Meetings Through Power Sharing." *Harvard Business Review* 50, no. 4 (July-August 1972): 47-54.

Reichman, W. and Levy, M. "Psychological Restraints on Effective Planning." *Management Review* 64, no. 10 (October 1975): 37-42.

Scott, William. "The Creative Individual." *Journal of the Academy of Management* 8, no. 3 (Sept. 1965): 211-219.

American Hospital Association. "Statement of the Governing Board and Planning." in *The Practice of Planning in Health Care Institutions*. Chicago: American Hospital Association, 1973:87.

American Hospital Association. "Statement on the Physician and Planning." in *The Practice of Planning in Health Care Institutions*. Chicago: American Hospital Association, 1973.

Chapter 3

Organizing for Planning

To carry out his responsibilities for planning, the chief executive will have to see to it that the work of planning is accomplished in a competent manner. He will need to consider if he can coordinate and guide the planning function, or to what extent he should delegate this to others. The planning role of the chief executive will vary with the size of his organization; and, as with his other management functions, some point will be reached when he needs planning help. A formal planning program will require the lavish use of time, but lack of time should not be used as an excuse to neglect the process. A well-organized planning process cannot be installed in a health organization overnight with immediate results. Much time and patience is necessary to produce a worthwhile and workable long range plan and to keep it up to date.

THE WORK OF PLANNING

Much of this book is devoted to discussions of planning work. Before choosing an organizational structure for planning, the chief executive should want to review the kind of work that will need to be accomplished. Table 3.1 lists the work required in the health facility planning function.

There is no single way for the health facility's chief executive to discharge his responsibilities for the planning function. Major problems that often stand in the way are the shortage of time, lack of appropriate temperament, and a myriad of other operating problems that must be resolved.[1]

Table 3.1

WORK OF THE HEALTH FACILITY PLANNING FUNCTION

1. Organize a formal planning process involving the right people with the right information to make recommendations on the future of the institution.
2. Stimulate the effective development of formal planning among each of the divisions and departments and integrate their plans with overall institutional plans.
3. Study the institution's current programs of service, the nature of the communities served by those programs, and their relationship to the programs of other health care institutions serving the same area.
4. Identify community gaps in service and opportunities for program innovations, and recommend allocations of institutional resources for new or existing programs.
5. Establish planning links with other health institutions and agencies, and identify and evaluate opportunities for joint or shared programs of service.
6. Continually survey evolving trends in economic, political, and social characteristics of the community served; and recommend actions to advance the institution's ability to be responsive to community needs.
7. Guide an organized process of institutional goal evaluation and development, and coordinate the development of strategies for achieving the institution's objectives.
8. Maintain an appropriate follow-up program of progress made on decisions resulting from planning activites.

FORMS OF PLANNING ORGANIZATION

There is no universal or best arrangement for organizing to do the work of planning. The planning function is related so intimately to the entire management process and organizational structure that each form evolves and is influenced by particular institutional characteristics. The nature and scope of a health institution will affect the requirements for planning as will the personality of the chief executive. One chief executive might want to do his own planning regardless of hospital size; at the other extreme, another might prefer to operate by involving more people in planning work. Previous success or failure with planning can greatly influence its organizational form in an institution, as will the amount of experience there has been with the process.[2]

The organizational patterns usually take one of the following forms (see Fig. 3.1):

1. No formal planning program exists at all. Planning is done by each line manager in conjunction with the annual budgeting cycle or as needed for new projects. In the case of modernization or expansion projects, planning might be carried out by a consultant to demonstrate feasibility and help in securing approvals by outside agencies.

2. A personal assistant to the chief executive is assigned the responsibility. His duties can include other aspects of the organization, but a major focus is on planning "staff work." This can include collecting and evaluating data, writing position papers, and providing staff. assistance to planning groups. In such cases, the chief executive often is the central focal point for planning, with his assistant providing aid where needed. In some situations the staff assistant assumes greater responsibility to represent the chief executive.

3. A line manager's assignments are organized to permit him time to carry out the job. Although he can be responsible for other functional areas, a portion of his time will be spent on planning work. He might or might not serve as a planning focal point depending on the wishes of the chief executive.

4. An executive vice president or president is responsible for all planning, and an operating chief executive is responsible to him for current operations. The top planning individual usually will have staff assistance to help him carry out this function.

5. A planning executive and staff are made the central focus for all planning work, with that individual reporting to the chief executive officer. The responsibilities of this department can encompass the entire planning function, including liaison with outside agencies and project management in the case of expansion or modernization.

6. In multi-institutional systems a variation of the previous form includes a planning executive or staff in each major division or operating unit, with overall system planning the responsibility of a planning officer at central headquarters.

Figure 3.1

FORMS OF PLANNING ORGANIZATIONS

Chief Executive's Personal Assistant

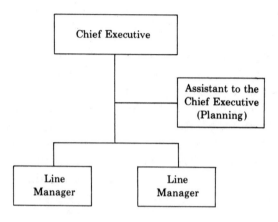

Partial Responsibility of a Line Manager

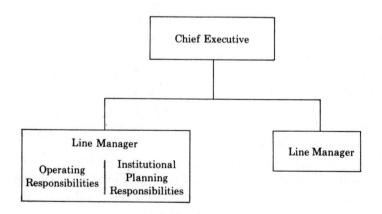

Executive Vice President Delegates Operations

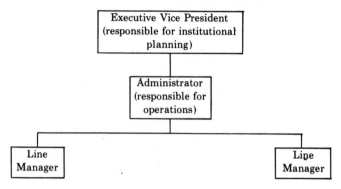

Director of Planning and Staff

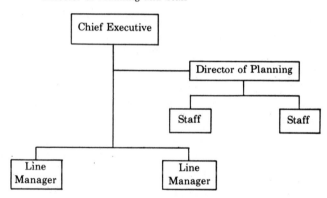

Multi-institutional System Planning

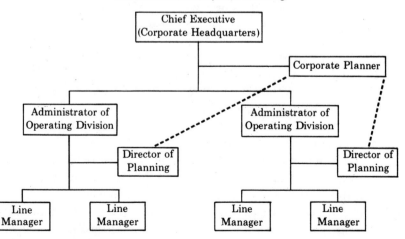

SHOULD A HEALTH INSTITUTION HAVE A PLANNING DEPARTMENT?

Among the planning arrangements becoming more frequently employed by larger health institutions is the planning department, directed by an individual who reports to the chief executive. The advantages of having a competent staff focus full-time on the planning work previously described have become realized by a number of organizations, especially those with rapidly changing communities, heightened competition for physicians and community support, uncertain futures, and strong outside regulations.

However, planning departments are expensive, and institutional resources are limited. Not every facility will be able to acquire the full-time planning help they need. Some institutions, especially those in one-hospital towns, might not feel the pressure to employ other than minimal planning assistance. Others are directed by chief executives wishing to remain the strong central planning focus, although the existence of a planning department does not automatically imply a lessening of chief executive prerogatives: to the contrary, if a planning department is used as an excuse to avoid top management's planning responsibilities, it probably should not be created.

Planning departments are also not without organizational problems. The age-old problems of defining line and staff prerogatives and developing constructive relationships are especially present in the planning function. A planning department removed from operations or one that attempts to do all the planning will receive uncooperative support from those on the line. Planning requires the active involvement of those who will be held responsible for plan implementation. The lack of line involvement and commitment to the process has doomed many well-conceived plans to failure. Yet this tendency to separate planning from operations often becomes more pronounced where a formal planning department exists. Since planning is a prime function of every manager and the process is wrapped up in the entire decision-making apparatus, a separate planning department can create an unnatural division of responsibilities. When creating a planning department, therefore, care must be taken to build in a formal line involvement and provision for the planner's responsibility for judging his success by whether plans are implemented.

The technique of evaluating planning by success in implementation implies a great deal about an institutional planner's qualifications and how he carries out his job. Although actual implementation is normally carried out by an organization's operating managers, the planner has a responsibility to propose plans that are workable. This means that not only will physical, human, and financial resources be available, but also that those who implement are psychologically prepared to devote their time and energy to the process.

QUALIFICATIONS OF THE INSTITUTIONAL PLANNER

A list of personal specifications for a health institution planner would include a group of qualifications that could be applied equally to most other top staff positions in an organization. One such list, borrowed from corporate planning, indicates that he should be

1. mature in bearing and attitude
   - emotionally well adjusted,
   - commanding in demeanor and actions,
   - sufficiently self-assured to take strong stands when warranted;
2. willing to recommend calculated risks to improve the company
   - able to cut new patterns,
   - willing to break out of conventional methods,
   - willing to generate innovation and depart from conventional ways of doing things;
3. highly intelligent and creative
   - capable of analyzing business and economic problems involving all aspects of the business and arriving at sound conclusions;
4. tactful and persuasive
   - able to deal effectively with both operating and senior executive

- willing to help operating executives with specific planning problems
5. in excellent health
   - able and willing to devote his time and energies to the demanding requirements of the position[3]

How a health institution planner carries out his job is a chief factor responsible for whether the planning process will be successful. He should never give the impression that he makes planning decisions, but rather that he needs to "sell" his views to line management. His influence and persuasiveness in the organization must be based on his knowledge and abilities, not on his proximity to the chief executive's office. "Authority" has little application as a tool of the institutional planner. He needs to be flexible and open-minded in his relationships with others in the organization and must seek to achieve compromise and the understanding of views between parties. Sound planning requires sound and reliable data, but the planner should not get so engrossed in details and justifications that management actions become unreasonably delayed. Management intuition and judgment should be sharpened by planning and planning data, not stifled by information requirements. The planner should be a catalyst for the creation of innovative plans by management and the medical staff. He should create a climate where others seek his advice, data, analytical abilities, and objectivity. Obviously, to accomplish the above, the planner's human relations skills should be impeccable; he should be able to communicate well both in writing and orally. He certainly needs to be psychologically well balanced and to be able to cope with the frustrations inherent in the job. Of course, one realizes that these personal characteristics are valuable for most responsible management positions.

⚜ PLANNING COMMITTEES

The need for maximum involvement in the institutional planning process necessitates the creation of groups of individuals who can effectively channel diverse opinion into common action. Already mentioned is the "planning committee" of the governing body, which formalizes the commitment of that group and focuses the ultimate responsibility for planning decisions. This should be a standing committee, chaired by a respected member of the board who will encourage and not thwart discussion and debates. The function of this committee will be to study the institution's external and internal environments, evaluate alternative courses of both short range and long range action, understand the implications on those who will be affected by those actions, make recommendations to its parent organization, and establish a mechanism to evaluate continuously past plans in light of changing environments. The process is obviously cyclical, requiring a continuously functioning planning committee, well guided by clearly focused issues, appropriate information, and knowledgeable input.

By composition the board planning committee should include a membership that balances the views of the board, medical staff, administration, and other key groups both inside and outside the institution. Some of its members might be appointed by nature of their office or position, and others might be elected by their constituencies.

The individual who is responsible for the planning function should serve as staff to this committee and work closely with the chairman in the development of agenda, dissemination of material to members, presentation of position papers, provision of knowledgeable opinion, and action behind the scenes to achieve consensus. Committee meetings should be well prepared, with background materials circulated well in advance of a scheduled meeting. Because of the broad scope of subjects that will encompass the committee's charge and the divergence of opinion and perspectives of its members, lack of work structure and organization can result in endless deliberations with little substance.

The board's planning committee serves as the central focus for channeling the opinions, proposals, and suggestions of the organization and the many publics served by the institution. Appropriate mechanisms should, therefore, be structured to allow a free exchange of opinion and the opportunity for potentially useful ideas to reach the top planning body. Such ideas could emerge from the medical staff, nursing staff, other employees, community groups, other institutions, or outside agencies.

A particularly good example of this process was observed in a 300-bed community hospital in a large city in Pennsylvania. The hospital has been experimenting for about a year with the process for getting effective input into planning decisions from both internal and external groups. The medical staff had complained that historically their views had not been sought on major planning decisions that were made by an "elite group of board members." The medical staff as a whole was "demanding" a bigger role in the management of the institution. Likewise, community groups were seeking greater involvement in health industry decisions and were getting it through federal legislation mandating their participation on the boards of comprehensive health planning agencies. To respond to these pressures for participatory planning, the hospital created a management planning committee, medical staff planning committee, and a community advisory committee to serve this function (see Fig. 3.2). These groups not only passed on their ideas and proposals to the board committee but also reviewed and commented on the conclusions or recommendations of the board with respect to planning options. The management planning group was composed of the entire administrative staff and key department heads. This group was chaired by the administrator and staffed by an institutional planner, who in that institution was an assistant administrator with duties arranged so he could carry out this function. This committee served as an important link between the entire employee organization and the board planning committee.

The Medical Staff Planning Committee was created by the organized medical staff with its members appointed by their elected president. The committee's charge as written in the staff bylaws was to "serve as a focus for planning ideas or proposals emerging from the medical staff and evaluate options for institutional development in terms of impact on the medical staff. Its charge also included the provision of knowledgeable input into the design of any new programs or facilities." The committee was chaired by a member of the staff who was appointed by the medical staff president. Staffing the committee and attending all its meetings was the Assistant Administrator for Planning.

The Community Advisory Committee was created specifically to channel the ideas and opinions of the important external

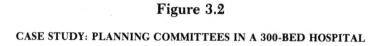

Figure 3.2

CASE STUDY: PLANNING COMMITTEES IN A 300-BED HOSPITAL

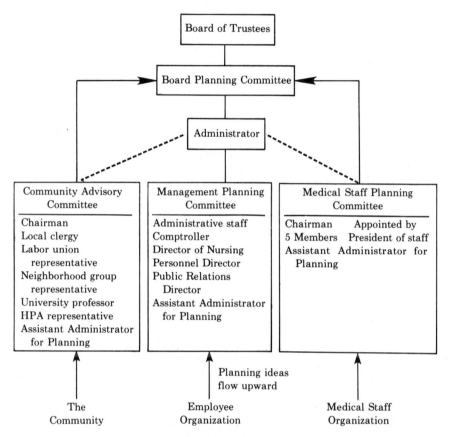

public served by the institution. By composition the committee membership included local clergy, a labor union representative, neighborhood group representatives, a professor from the local university, and a representative from the local HSA. The chairman was one of the members of the clergy, and he was provided staff assistance by the Assistant Administrator for Planning. The committee often invited other members of the community to their meetings to hear their views on important planning issues and discuss the implications of new community and institutional developments. Careful records were kept of minutes and statements made to the committee, and a report was made at each

monthly meeting of the board planning committee by the community group chairman, who also served as a member of the top
planning group.

A common thread throughout the committee planning structure
is the "institutional planner," who gives continuity to the process
and makes sure that the right hand knows what the left hand is
doing. In the above case, he was the Assistant Administrator for
Planning. He is the one individual who can see the entire process
in perspective and can coordinate committee deliberations so the
process can move forward in a timely manner. He can detect immediately when actions taken by two different committees are
contradictory and can seek to resolve differences or disputes
before they become issues for open debate at the board planning
level. The time that obviously must be devoted to this coordination function clearly supports the need for full-time commitment
on the part of one individual.

It is important that the organization maintain confidence in the
planning committee's ability to deal effectively with planning
problems. The committee should work toward demonstrating
tangible results of its planning efforts. It is easy to get bogged
down with endless discussions of past problems or unrelated
issues. The need to experience early success to help create a
favorable "planning climate" was discussed in a previous section.
Providing deliberate well-thought-out staff support to the committee is one way to influence meaningful outcomes. An effective
chairman who is skilled in achieving closure will further help
assure constructive meetings.

Much of the literature on the functions of the board planning
committee suggests that its work should begin with an examination of the institution's goals. In many institutions this has proven
to be a very difficult and painful process, opening up a Pandora's
box of strongly held values and notions and seemingly unending
debate on basic institutional philosophy. In such a "planning climate" it is difficult, at best, to achieve early success by demonstrating tangible results of the process. On the contrary, if not constrained, the process could appear to be destroying the organization.

At some time, however, the committee will have to evaluate critically institutional goals and the implications of those goals on

future actions and programs, no matter how painful the process. Some committees have been able to breeze through the goal-setting process with limited confrontation, especially when outside events were challenging institutional survival. A later section of this book will discuss this extremely important goal-setting process, which can more rationally follow an objective analysis of both the external and internal planning environments, the subject of the next chapter.

SUMMARY

There is no one best way to organize for planning or carry out the work required. Much will depend on the time and temperament of the chief executive officer. The work of planning usually requires considerable effort to assure that it is carried out competently. Information must be collected, analyzed, and reported. Individuals and groups have to be educated, cajoled, and persuaded. Planning by various internal and external groups has to be linked effectively. And a program of follow-up, evaluation, and adjustment must be continuously monitored. Most institutions have found that the chief executive has to delegate much of the work of planning while still maintaining the overall responsibility for the results. A variety of organizational forms are available for examination, but the form chosen will greatly depend on the organization, the capabilities of its top management personnel, patterns of delegation and authority, and the history of planning within the institution.

The important consideration is that a formal planning structure should be created to channel diverse opinion and activities effectively into common actions. To give everyone a piece of that action, a structure of committees is usually created to represent the interests of the governing body, management, medical staff, employees, and the community. Properly staffing each of these committees is an essential ingredient, as is guiding and linking their individual efforts into a common direction. The risk of indecision and endless debate among diverse groups is great if a deliberate effort is not taken to organize and provide a planning structure to guide the process.

Notes

1. For a good review of the work involved in planning see *The Practice of Planning in Health Care Institutions* (Chicago: American Hospital Association, 1973).

2. For a discussion of how one medical center formed conclusions on how to organize its planning program see Phil Goodwin, "Why One Hospital Implemented a Formal Planning System and How It Works Today," *Hospital Financial Management* (February 1975), pp. 20-23.

3. George Steiner, *Top Management Planning* (Toronto, Ontario: MacMillan Company, 1969), p. 128.

Suggested References

American Hospital Association. *The Practice of Planning in Health Care Institutions.* Chicago: American Hospital Association, 1973.

Goodwin, P. "Why One Hospital Implemented a Formal Planning System and How It Works Today." *Hospital Financial Management* 29, no. 2 (Feb. 1975): 20-23.

Gordon, P. and Harvey, J. "The Intra Institutional Planning Process." *Hospital Administration* 14, no. 4 (Fall 1969).

Litochect, R.J. "The Structure of Long Range Planning Groups." *Journal of the Academy of Management* 14, no. 1 (March 1971): 53-58.

Steiner, George A. *Top Management Planning.* Toronto, Ontario: MacMillan Company, 1969.

Warren, Kirby E. *Long Range Planning: The Executive Viewpoint.* Englewood Cliffs, N.J.: Prentice Hall, Inc., 1966.

Webber, J.B. and Dula, M.A. "Effective Planning Committees for Hospitals." *Harvard Business Review* 52, no. 3 (May-June 1974): 133-142.

Chapter 4

Analyzing the External Environment

To establish a clear framework upon which to base decisions on an institution's role and its short and long range goals, the planning committee needs to become knowledgeable about external and internal factors that will have an impact on the nature of the institution. A planning committee armed with this knowledge can address both the probable future opportunities for institutional development and the environmental problems that might constrain future actions. The committee should not only be concerned with the impact of the environment on the institution but also the impact of the institution on the environment, for the latter will affect the future environment for planning.

COMMUNITY SURVEY

The amount of statistical data that can be collected about the institution's external environments is beyond that which any serious institutional planner can put to practical use. The planning literature abounds with descriptions of how to conduct community surveys and the data requirements for such studies. An outline of one approach is shown below.

I.   Demographic characteristics
  1. Population size
  2. Age distribution
  3. Sex ratio
  4. Marital status
  5. Ethnic and cultural characteristics
  6. Education levels

       7. Economic status
       8. Population density
       9. Degree of urbanization
     10. Racial composition

II.   Ecological characteristics
      1. Housing and living conditions
      2. Water supply and waste disposal
      3. Transportation and travel times
      4. Land usage
      5. Zoning
      6. Urban renewal
      7. Topography
      8. Governmental structure
      9. Industrial development

III. Community health status
      1. Positive measurements
         a. Birth rates
         b. Fertility rates
         c. Life expectancy
      2. Negative measurements
         a. Mortality
            i. Crude death rate
           ii. Age specific death rate
         b. Morbidity
            i. Incidence of disease
           ii. Prevelence of disease
           iii. Disability data
      3. Social well being
         a. Divorce
         b. Desertion
         c. Alcoholism
         d. Drug abuse
         e. Crime and delinquency
         f. Illegitimacy
         g. Prostitution
         h. Mental illness

    4.   Social pathology
       a. Unemployment
       b. Poverty and deprivation
       c. Illiteracy
       d. Existence of basic community services[1]

Not included in the above listing is information about the community health system itself, including numbers, types, and location of health manpower, health institutions and agencies, and the scope of existing services. One such listing, based on the objective of facilities and levels of care, is as follows:

I.   Facilities for care of ambulatory patients
    A.   Physicians', dentists', or other practitioners' offices
       1. Solo
       2. Associated group
       3. Organized group
    B.   Hospital clinics—general or special
    C.   Health department clinics
    D.   Industrial clinics
    E.   School clinics
    F.   Other clinics
    G.   Rehabilitation centers
    H.   Neighborhood service centers
    I.   Community mental health centers
II. Facilities for emergency services
    A.   First aid stations
    B.   Emergency service units
       1. Community-based
       2. Hospital-based
III. Facilities for patients requiring residential care (in-patient)
    A.   Short term general hospitals
    B.   Short term special hospitals
    C.   Chronic disease and long term hospitals
    D.   Acute psychiatric hospitals
    E.   General hospital sections of psychiatric communities
    F.   Rehabilitation hospitals
    G.   Extended care facilities

H.   Nursing homes
   1.   Skilled
   2.   Intermediate
I.   Infirmaries
   1.   Schools and colleges
   2.   Sections of homes for the aged and homes for children

IV.   Facilities for organized home care services
   A.   Comprehensive
      1.   Community-based
      2.   Hospital-based
   B.   Visiting nurse agencies

V.   Facilities for supporting services
   A.   Pharmacies
   B.   Clinical laboratories
   C.   Dental laboratories
   D.   Radiology services
   E.   Ambulance stations
   F.   Prosthesis and appliance fitters and makers
   G.   Opticians

VI.   Supply services
   A.   Manufacturers and distributors of drugs
   B.   Manufacturers and distributors of medical and dental supplies and equipment
   C.   Publishers of health services literature[2]

Reproduced with permission of the editor from *Health Planning Qualitative Aspects and Qualitative Techniques.*

The degree of detail with which the nature of the external environment can be assessed is limited only by ingenuity, money, and the availability of information. *A more important consideration for any institution is whether the data will be useful in making planning decisions.* The institutional planning committee has to determine which information is applicable to decisions that have to be made, which is most important, which should receive in-depth study, and how much money and manpower should be spent in the process. A large number of health institutions have spent thousands of dollars for comprehensive community surveys, only to find that much of the data they paid to have collected were never used to define or project the institution's future.

There is no formula to tell an institutional planning group what external forces to analyze and how much time and money to devote to the process. What is essential, however, is that they know what kinds of questions need to be asked and what impact the answers to those questions are likely to have on the future of the institution. The kinds of questions asked in planning suggest the type of data and quantitative analysis required. The importance or impact of each question provides a frame for deciding on the time and money that should be devoted to seeking answers.[3]

To illustrate the difference between high and low impact questions consider the following situation that faced North Hospital, a 400-bed acute care hospital in a large southern city. Established thirty years ago to meet the needs of a defined Catholic population, the hospital has witnessed a changing local community, population shifts to the suburbs, and a deterioriation of its local neighborhood and community support. An out-migration of middle income families and replacement by disadvantaged groups has changed the service needs of the local population and has caused considerable shifting of physician loyalties toward more suburban health facilities.

In an area approximately one square mile are three major health facilities in addition to North Hospital. There is a 568-bed full service institution which is now completing a $20 million modernization program making it the largest medical facility in the area. A proprietary institution, with a bed complement of 196, is operated by a major hospital chain as a basic medical/surgical institution. A little more than two years ago this proprietary hospital added 100 beds in a new addition. The University Medical Center operates a 180-bed full service teaching facility. With the recent appointment of a new dean of the College of Medicine it has been rumored that some planning is underway to examine the possibilities of adding a new teaching facility on a site adjacent to the college campus.

Within this environment, competition for physicians, patients, and new programs has been intense, with few examples of cooperative planning. As an example, recently each of the institutions applied for, justified, and gained approval to purchase an EMI scanner with no notable efforts to explore sharing arrangements. Clearly, in order to remain viable, North Hospital must focus its long range planning on what future role it will play in this intensively competitive medical marketplace.

There are also a number of immediate pressures facing the institution's decision makers.

- The hospital has been experiencing increasing demands for services, particularly in the medical and surgical programs which have been operating at nearly 100 percent occupancy.

- A number of hospital departments are functioning in crowded conditions. Those that have been identified as being critically short of space are the laboratories, radiology, physical therapy, education, inhalation therapy, EEG, and EKG.

- The hospital's site is extremely constrained, with limited space for horizontal expansion and little available parking accommodations.

- As both community and governmental pressures increase the demand for ambulatory care services, the hospital faces the need to expand or alter its outpatient facilities.

- The need for an on-site professional office building has been a pressing issue that must be considered in light of the effect such a building may have on admission practices.

Considering this limited picture, Table 4.1 presents examples of the high versus low impact planning questions to be raised by such an institution.

Although the low impact statements listed above indeed could have some importance in dealing with the issues at hand, in the situation described the institution would not want to devote considerable monies to their detailed analysis. For example, the question of evaluating the political power structure could take an expensive study of considerable sophistication. However, a municipal hospital seeking to increase its political influence and community support could require a detailed study of how the community power structure is changing, and how those changes will impact the institution.

Table 4.1

HIGH AND LOW IMPACT QUESTIONS

High

1. What population does this institution serve, and how has it been changing?
2. Is the present mission of the institution relevant to the needs of the population it serves?
3. Is the institution willing to commit itself to offer new programs or services to presently served groups? What are those program needs?
4. Is the institution prepared to make changes in structure, programs, or facilities to reach new population groups?

Low

1. What is the pattern of government in this community and the political power structure?
2. What are the leading causes of death and disease by census tract?
3. What are the institution's research needs and capabilities?

Communities also vary in the extent to which needed information is available and the form in which it can be collected. One area might have a detailed computer printout of some informational need; another might require a complete data collection and processing job. The implications on information costs of these two situations should be obvious. Given the cost and time constraints placed on the planning process, therefore, answering the same question in different institutions can result in different levels of data sophistication and analysis.

HIGH IMPACT QUESTIONS ABOUT THE COMMUNITY

Health facilities engaged in a comprehensive planning program will find that there are a number of high impact questions about the external environment common to most situations. The following discussion centers on the nature of these questions and their importance to an institution.

What population does the institution serve, and how is it changing in size or composition? What will the impact of these changes be on the institution?

The history of most health care institutions is an account of organizational adaptations to changing service populations. Increases or decreases in population size, changes the overall demand for health services. Shifts of that population into the suburbs, for example, can raise serious questions about the future of an inner city hospital. When those shifts are accompanied by significant changes in social or economic makeup, other questions are raised about types of services and how they will be financed. A great deal of health services are age related (for example, obstretrics and pediatrics). Therefore, changing age composition of a population will have considerable influence on program needs. Population groups can be dissected into detailed age cohorts, ethnic groups, educational levels, income levels, occupational characteristics, and other variables; but unless these data are used in planning decisions they probably are not worth collecting.

To find out what population the institution serves, the most common technique is to conduct a patient origin study. Simply stated, this technique involves the analysis of a sample of patient discharges by place of residence to determine what communities are most important to the institution. If one asks the reverse question, "to which communities is the institution most important," some different kinds of answers usually emerge. The second type of study requires the compilation of patient origin data from all other health facilities serving the same population area. Information on discharges from other institutions is often difficult to obtain if there is no community agency granted the authority to collect and disseminate these data. Even where such an agency exists, some institutions might not have participated in the information-sharing program. Such will not be the case under the envisioned HSA planning, and health institutions should benefit from the availability of more comprehensive planning information.

The results of the former type of study show the percentage of the patient population in each community served by your institution. Using both techniques, many institutions find that some communities might only account for a small percentage of their patients yet look to that institution as a sole or major provider of health services. Most institutions have different service areas for the various services they provide and should consider these differences when projecting future program needs. For example, a hospital's primary service area for emergency care could be a population residing within a five-mile radius or perhaps a fifteen-minute drive to the facility, whereas its service area for kidney dialysis could be the whole region.

To illustrate how these service area studies are typically conducted the following example is provided.

Community Hospital is a 167-bed general acute care facility located in the center of Walnut County, which had a 1975 population of 71,500. The hospital historically has drawn a large number of its patients from counties adjacent to Walnut namely Henry, Gordon, Bruce, and Frank, which had a combined population of 123,600 in 1975. Service area analysis was initiated by abstracting patient residence information from the records of all patients discharged during the most recent twelve-month period and coding these data by geographic areas of the city, as shown in Table 4.2. To relate these data to geographic location and proximity to Community Hospital, a map of Walnut County postal zones is shown in Figure 4.1.

An analysis of this information revealed that 20.3 percent of the patients discharged during the period resided in the area adjacent to the hospital (Zip Code Zone 30001). Community Hospital's primary service area was composed of Center City (Zip Code Zones 30001, 30002, 30003), Henry County, Bruce County, Gordon County, and Entertown (Zip Code Zones 30012, 30013, and 30014).[4] During the period 78.2 percent of the patients discharged resided in these areas. Residents of Frank County and Zip Code Zones 30004, 30005, 30008, and 30010, the secondary service area, comprised an additional 10.8 percent of the discharges. A comparative examination of discharge data from the period December 1970 to December 1973 revealed that this primary service area had changed little since 1971. Not only had the general service area not changed, but also the percent of discharges attributable to its component regions had also remained relatively stable. The only change noted was a slight drop in the percentage of discharges from Allentown and a concomitant slight increase in the percentage of discharges from Entertown. Although the percentage of discharges for residents of Center City and out-of-county residents remained the same over this period, it appeared that the

Figure 4.1

MAP OF WALNUT COUNTY
(with postal zones)

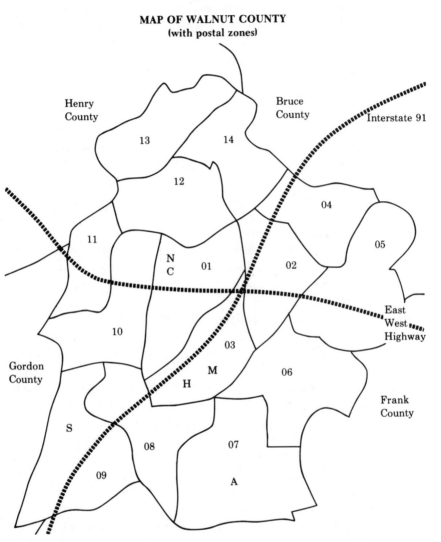

		Communities	Zones
C — Community Hospital	N — Northern University	Center City	01,02,03
M — Memorial Hospital	H — Health Department	Allentown	04,05
S — Suburban Hospital	01-14 — (Postal Zone)	Birchville	06,07
A — Air Force Hospital		Chester	08,09
		Downville	10,11
		Entertown	12,13,14

slight shift noted in other regions within the service area merely were reflective of the population flow within the county.

While the patient origin study indicated the importance of geographic areas to Community Hospital, a study of Community's share of the market in each of the areas revealed how much the residents of those areas rely on Community to meet their hospitalization needs. The results of such a study based on discharges during calendar year 1975 are furnished in Table 4.3.

This table also compares the patient origin study to the share of the market study. An analysis of this information revealed several important factors. In several of the areas that contribute heavily to Community's workload, a large percentage of the residents used other Walnut County Hospitals. This is especially true of Gordon County and Zip Code Zones 30002 and 30003, and to a lesser extent of Bruce County and Zip Code Zone 30001. This in-

Table 4.2

PATIENT ORIGIN STUDY—1975
FOR COMMUNITY HOSPITAL

Patient Residences Zone or County	Number of Discharges	Percent of Total Discharges	Cumulative Percent of Total Discharges
30001	998	20.3%	20.3%
Henry	500	10.1	30.4
Bruce	450	9.1	39.5
Gordon	420	8.5	48.0
30003	375	7.6	55.6
30002	352	7.2	62.8
30013	270	5.5	68.3
30012	260	5.3	73.6
30014	225	4.6	78.2
30004	175	3.6	81.8
Frank	150	3.1	84.9
30005	105	2.1	87.0
30008	72	1.5	88.5
30010	72	1.5	90.0
30006	70	1.4	91.4
30009	41	0.8	92.2
30007	40	0.8	93.0
30011	33	0.7	93.7
Other	304	6.2	99.9

dicates the need for coordinated action by Community Hospital and other facilities in meeting the needs of these population groups. Second, it is noted that Community is the major source of hospitalization in several of the geographic areas in which reside a relatively small percentage of Community Hospital's patients. For example, during the study period only 4.6 percent of Community's patient discharges resided in Zip Code Zone 30014, but 81.8 percent of all patients hospitalized from this zone were treated at Community. Therefore certain areas with a relatively low population count rely heavily on Community for hospital services, even though those areas do not individually account for a large percentage of the hospital's workload.

Following this general review of its service area, Community Hospital further analyzed its discharge data for patient origin by major service including medical, surgical, obstetrics, pediatrics,

Table 4.3

SHARE OF THE MARKET ANALYSIS

Patient Residence by Zone of County	Number of Discharges in Walnut Hospitals	Each hospital's percent of total discharges for areas of residence:				Percent of Community's Total Discharges
		Suburban	Memorial	Air Force	Community	
30001	1468	1.3%	30.6%	—	67.9%	20.3%
30002	1202	2.0	68.6	—	29.2	7.2
30003	1130	4.8	61.9	—	33.1	7.6
30004	270	9.2	25.9	—	64.8	3.6
30005	175	5.7	34.2	—	60.0	2.1
30006	646	2.3	42.5	44.2	10.8	1.4
30007	1550	2.2	14.5	80.6	2.5	0.8
30008	563	81.8	5.3	—	12.7	1.5
30009	536	88.6	3.7	—	7.6	0.8
30010	249	64.2	6.8	—	28.9	1.5
30011	100	52.0	15.0	—	33.0	0.7
30012	319	15.6	2.8	—	81.5	5.3
30013	350	19.1	3.7	—	77.1	5.5
30014	275	13.4	4.7	—	81.8	4.6
Henry	542	4.2	3.5	—	92.2	10.1
Gordon	990	55.5	2.0	—	42.4	8.5
Bruce	611	15.7	10.6	—	73.6	9.1
Frank	372	38.1	21.5	—	40.3	3.1
Other	367	11.7	5.4	—	82.8	6.2

emergency, and other outpatient services. This analysis confirmed, for example, that the hospital served as a regional referral center for pediatric inpatient services.

But knowledge of a health institution's geographic areas of service is only a first step in planning for the future health service needs of people. How the population served will change in size and composition and the implication of those changes on their health needs is a crucial question to be answered in planning for future hospital programs. However, projections of population and their characteristics are only as good as the assumptions upon which they are based. Differing assumptions, for example, about birth and death rates, migration patterns, and industrial and community developments will result in varying projections of relatively equal validity. But this inherent uncertainty about the future should not be used as an excuse to forego planning. Rather, it points out the need for periodic reassessment of an institution's assumptions about its future environment and its flexibility to revise plans as required.

How will the population served utilize the institution's programs and services?

The utilization of a health facility's services, or a community's health services, for that matter, is the result of a complex set of factors related to how people translate their actual health needs into effective demand. Projecting how a given population will utilize an institution's health services is often one of the most awesome tasks facing the institutional planner. To illustrate the complexity of this job, consider projecting the future use of an institution's chronic kidney disease program. Lets trace the steps that a patient takes before he actually arrives at the hospital's door.

1. Patient develops a diseased kidney. The prevelence of the disease can be affected by a variety of environmental, genetic, and social factors. Significant changes in pollution control, genetic counseling, or social well being in a community could impact the number of cases found in the population.

2. Patient recognizes symptoms and seeks help. Both the recognition of symptoms and an individual's response can vary con-

siderably among different population groups due to a number of factors including educational levels, cultural determinants, and attitudes toward ill health and the belief that a health professional can effect a cure. Significant changes in any of these factors can greatly increase the tendency to seek professional help for the disease at its early stages.

3. Physician diagnoses a chronic kidney disease. Accurate diagnosis could depend on the existence of properly trained physicians and their availability to the population. Advances in medical technology bring better diagnostic techniques for more accurate and timely identification of the disease.

4. Prognosis calls for hospital admission and treatment. But the patient must accept the treatment as prescribed. He could delay an immediate response due to an attitude about hospitals, problems in getting assistance in caring for family members, or the fear of income loss during time away from work. If he has no private health insurance coverage for such care, and if he is not eligible for government assistance, the delay in getting proper care could be extended, or even fatal.

5. Patient is admitted to the hospital. This assumes that a hospital is available and will accept his admission, considering financial resources and insurance coverage. It also assumes that the patient's physician has privileges at that institution. If no hospital is easily accessible to the patient, or if none of the existing hospitals provide the services needed, then a long drive could provide a further barrier to receiving timely care. The use of a distant hospital's services will not show up in the use rate of the hospitals in the patient's community, which further complicates the measurement of community demand for this service.

This process was an exaggerated example to show the variety of complex factors that can affect the actual utilization of a specific health service within a community.[5] Yet, projecting utilization is a basic prerequisite, to properly sizing hospital programs and facilities required to house these programs. The most common resolution to this problem is to simplify the analysis by projecting future demand on the basis of historical use rates and multiplying these rates by the anticipated population at risk. For example, in the case of future demand for obstetrical services, we might use a forecast of the number of women between fourteen and forty-four and multiply by a projected fertility rate. Or we could simplify the process even more by projecting so many obstetrical beds needed per 1,000 population, as was the method used in the Hill-Burton program.*

Projecting future utilization on the basis of historical utilization, however, has inherent risks, namely that a significant change will occur in an underlying factor affecting the use of health services. Such was the case when the Medicare program went into effect. Few analysts properly forecasted the surge in demand, which resulted from the removal of the financial barrier for those aged sixty-five and older. It would appear, however, that a reasonable approach is to adjust past use rates by the most informed judgment available to the analyst on the forces that will change future use, and the links between the forces and utilization patterns.[6]

The actual utilization of an institution's health services, therefore, should be used to gauge future resource requirements only to the extent that answers to the following questions are analyzed.

1. Present use rates reflect the decisions of those members of the community who actually used health services. To what extent has that service been underutilized by the population due to one or more factors limiting individual understanding or access?

2. Is the use rate deflated as a result of care being delivered to the area's population by institutions outside the area? What factors are responsible for the out-migration for care, and will they be present in the future?

3. Is the use rate inflated due to specific attributes of the population, their insurance coverage, the practice of medicine in the area, or such? Will those factors continue to be responsible for overutilization in the future? For example, how will

---

* The Hospital Survey and Construction Act, P.L. 79-725, passed in August 1946, among other things, authorized grants to states for the purpose of surveying their needs and developing plans for the construction of health facilities.

utilization review and Professional Standards Review Organizations (PSROs) affect this overuse of a health service?

4. Is the rate inflated as a result of care being delivered by the area's health institutions to individuals from outside the area? What factors are responsible for the in-migration for care, and will they be present in the future? For example, will a new hospital in an area previously lacking one change those utilization patterns?

5. Does the institution anticipate outside pressures for change, or will it choose to initiate actions independently, which will either remove existing barriers or otherwise change utilization patterns? For example, a satellite clinic in a previously geographically isolated and medically underserved area could markedly affect future inpatient referrals. Or extending clinic hours to the evening might change the future volume of demand in the emergency room.

6. Which local, regional, or national trends or events will have an impact on future utilization rates—for example, national health insurance, a new breakthrough in medical technology, or stronger regulations or controls?

Current use rates should, therefore, be used cautiously in projecting future utilization. Answers to the above types of questions can help the analysts use rate adjustments to improve their reliability for future applications.

How is the nature of the community and its institutions changing, and what effect will these changes have on the health facility and its services?

Changing patterns of community life and services will have an impact on a health institution's planning. The structure of government and its political climate also can affect a health institution's influence in the community, as can the scope and nature of governmental and other social services. For example, a lax childhood immunization program will impact on the scope of pediatric facilities needed to cure preventable disease. An inadequate public transportation system might create a barrier to reaching needed health services by some population segments and could, in turn, suggest the need for institutional outreach services.

A community's industrial and business mix can also have a marked influence on a health facility. The occupational hazards associated with some industries will necessitate certain curative services. The expected growth or contraction of major companies can greatly affect future demands on a health facility, especially when it serves as a primary provider to those companies. The business mix and historical growth patterns will influence the stability of the community tax base, the availability of financing for social services, and the opportunities for philanthropy. Plans for city development, urban renewal, highway construction, business development, or rapid transit, for example, can have profound implications for the present and future development of a health facility.

One 300-bed general acute care hospital in the southeast was located in the suburbs of a large metropolitan area. One of the fastest growing counties of the state, the population grew between 1960 and 1970 by 128,799 or 61.7 percent. In 1960 that part of the county on the west bank of a major river had 36.3 percent of the entire county population. This portion increased to 37.3 percent by 1970. (In 1970 the west bank of the county accounted for 61.8 percent of the hospital's service area population.) Observers of population growth in the area concluded that the west bank population would continue to grow at a faster pace than that of the east bank for a number of reasons. First, the population density of the west bank was lower than that part of the county across the river, which is one of the older suburbs of the metropolitan area. On the west bank, large tracts of land were available for residential development. Because much of the metropolitan area's suburban growth as limited by natural geographic barriers, the west bank was expected to play an ever increasing role in absorbing the area's future suburban migration.

Critical to the institution's plans for future development, however, were assumptions about the growth in population over the next ten years. Reliable estimates were that the population of the area served by the hospital would double between 1975 and 1985. Yet, one critical assumption overrode all these growth estimates; that a new major high traffic bridge and expressway system will be built to link the area's future population with their jobs in the city. The bridge, which would cross the river, had been the subject of studies and debate for fifteen years with no resolution immediately in sight, chiefly because of political implications. There are strong pressures within the metropolitan government to thwart construction of the bridge to prevent further eroding of the center city's tax base by suburban flight. The construction of the bridge, and particularly its highway feeding network, is projected to have a significant impact on the character and integrity of a number of local communities, which have made strong appeals to their legislators. Future decisions on this issue will obviously have a profound effect on the future of this health facility.

What are the components of the community's health care system, how do they interrelate, and what projections or plans have been made for their development? How will anticipated changes in other components of the system impact on this health facility?

This question is analogous with a business seeking information about its competition, but here it includes the concept of evaluating opportunities for beneficial relationships between health facilities. Most health facilities coexist with other institutions or agencies that provide the same or complementary services. Changing populations or communities elicit different planning responses from these institutions depending on their perceptions of opportunities or threats, financial resources, and readiness to act. More than one health facility has seen a drastic change in the demand for specific services as a result of the planning actions of another institution. Likewise, two facilities attempting to provide the same services to a community (for example, pediatrics) might find that neither can do so efficiently or economically.

Which are the other health facilities that serve the same service communities? What are their strengths and weaknesses? What levels and types of services do they provide, and what formal agreements do they have with each other? What actions have they taken in the recent past, and what future developmental plans have been announced? Though the answers to these questions are often difficult to uncover, some educated judgments have to be made about how the future health care system structure will impact on institutional planning.

Most health facilities face an interesting paradox when evaluating their place in the community's health system. Concurrently with the need to be better at forecasting the future and leading new developments will be the pressure to share services and form joint arrangements with other institutions. Finding mutually beneficial joint institutional arrangements without giving up institutional prerogatives for adaptation and change is a difficult undertaking, especially for smaller facilities. The fear of domination of one institution over another is a very real one, posing serious roadblocks to many otherwise constructive arrangements.[7]

What are the community's long range HSPs, short range AIPs, and the implications for planning by this institution?

The National Health Planning Resources and Development Act requires a Health Systems Agency (HSA) to prepare a health systems plan (HSP) and an annual implementation plan (AIP) for the communities within its jurisdiction. Such plans will be based on an evaluation of a community's health needs, available health manpower, and resources. Projections will be made on the need for various kinds of health services, programs, and facilities; and priorities will be established for agency fund allocations.

The existence of such community health plans will create both opportunities and constraints for planning by a health facility. More information will be available about the health status and needs of a population. Groups of local community residents will determine how federal monies will be allocated to support needy projects. Health institutions will have much clearer guidelines by which to judge which of their programs are likely to receive strong community support. They will be encouraged to provide innovative approaches to health service delivery.

But, health facilities will be expected to conform with health plan priorities and develop institutional goals that complement community health goals. Desires by an institution to develop a more competitive program for a specific service could be thwarted in the name of duplication. Yet, the HSP will provide important information and guidelines for an institution engaging in an analysis of its external environment.

Occasionally a health institution might develop a long range plan or short term courses of action which are contrary to the guidelines and pronouncements of health planning bodies. One

250-bed hospital in the southeast studied the population it was serving and concluded that a fifty-bed expansion would be justified on the basis of population growth and the lack of alternative inpatient facilities. Service area analysis showed that a large number of people were going out of the immediate area to seek care because of this hospital's bed shortage and long waiting lists for admissions.

But the local planning agency had different ideas. Their analysis showed that within the geographic area under their jurisdiction, there were a sufficient number of beds to meet the population's needs for the next ten years. On this basis a moratorium was announced on new bed construction, and the agency refused to recommend this project under the review authority granted them by the state's certificate of need law. The matter was then taken to the courts, with the hospital challenging the methodology used by the planning agency in determining the population's need for beds. At issue was whether the bed need projection for an entire metropolitan area was an adequate basis for determining the needs of population groupings within that area. Or, approached another way, the hospital raised the question of how far should an individual have to travel for hospital care? The issue is still in litigation, but the point is that institutions should not be afraid to challenge community planning if it seems to them that it does not make sense.

HAZARDS OF PREDICTING THE FUTURE

One of the most important, and yet potentially the most hazardous, aspects of environmental analysis is the need to forecast the future. The present and future role of a hospital often is based on an analysis of historical utilization and a prediction of past trends in population, admissions, or service utilization.

A variety of techniques is used to analyze trends, some much more sophisticated than others. Often those results contradict rather than support each other. Trend analysis has an aura of sophistication and exactness that can result in misleading conclusions for the uninitiated. And yet so many conclusions about the future plans of an institution are based on some basic assumptions derived from projecting trend lines. Therefore, those responsible for an institution's long range planning process need to be discriminating users of trend projections and understand the limitations of the techniques used for their determination.

To illustrate the hazards of trend analysis consider the experience of one 300-bed community hospital in attempting to project obstetrical patient days based on historical utilization. Ten years of data were available, showing that patient days had declined from 12,195 in 1957 to 9,306 in 1966* (see Table 4.4). As part of a consultants study the number of obstetrical patient days to 1980 were projected under the assumption that the general movement of the historical data was downward in a linear fashion. The trend line was calculated by mathematically constructing the "best" straight line through the scatter of points. The results are shown in Table 4.5 and Figure 4.2.[8] Based on this analysis it was projected that the number of obstetrical patient days would continue to fall in a linear fashion to 4,330 days in 1980. The significance of this projection on the future utilization of facilities and, therefore, patient revenue would be significant.

The danger in this seemingly sophisticated projection is that, while a least squares linear trend can always be computed, the straight line might not make sense as a description of the underlying forces operating in the data. The trend might be considered as

Table 4.4

OBSTETRICAL PATIENT DAYS 1957—1966

Year	Actual Days
1957	12,195
1958	11,422
1959	10,397
1960	9,559
1961	9,004
1962	8,173
1963	9,034
1964	9,589
1965	9,122
1966	9,306

*While the data in this example may appear old, it has been purposely selected to compare what was projected with what actually happened.

a tendency for the data to increase or decrease over a long period of time. There is no implication that the increase or decrease is constant. It might be, of course; in which case the trend forms a straight line. But it could, in fact, follow complex curvilinear patterns.

Table 4.5

PROJECTED LINEAR TREND BY LEAST SQUARES METHOD

Year	Trend Value
1957	11,090
1958	10,800
1959	10,500
1960	10,210
1961	9,920
1962	9,620
1963	9,330
1964	9,030
1965	8,740
1966	8,450
Projected	
1967	8,150
1968	7,860
1969	7,560
1970	7,230
1971	6,700
1972	6,680
1973	6,390
1974	6,100
1975	5,800
1976	5,510
1977	5,210
1978	4,920
1979	4,630
1980	4,330

Another conceivable assumption would be that the historical data in our example followed a curvilinear pattern, with the decline of patient days reaching a bottom point in 1964, followed by an upswing that will continue through 1980. The method of least squares can also be used to fit the "best" curve through a scatter of points to construct a second degree trend line, as shown

Figure 4.2

GRAPH OF LINEAR TREND BY LEAST SQUARES METHOD

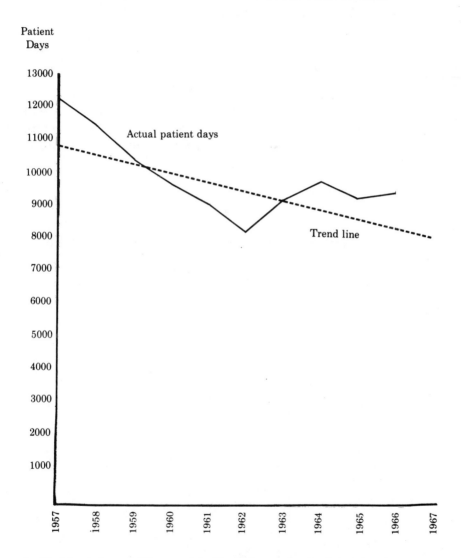

in Table 4.6 and Figure 4.3. By this method obstetrical patient days are projected to increase to 37,110 by 1980, which is 32,770 days greater than the number projected under the linear trend assumption.

Which projection is the correct one? On which trend should future requirements be based? Using a 75 percent occupancy level for obstetrics, projections for 1980 result in a forecasted bed need of sixteen at one extreme and 136 at the other. The potential financial impact of this decision is obvious.

Consider the Underlying Causes

Trend analysis provides projections of historical data under the assumption that the factors responsible for past patterns will have the same influence on future patterns of use. It is therefore important to understand the underlying causes of historical

Table 4.6

PROJECTED SECOND DEGREE TREND BY LEAST SQUARES METHOD

Year	Trend Values
1957	12,270
1958	11,180
1959	10,300
1960	9,620
1961	9,120
1962	8,830
1963	8,740
1964	8,830
1965	9,130
1966	9,630
1967	10,300
1968	11,200
1969	12,270
1970	13,550
1971	15,030
1972	16,690
1973	18,560
1974	20,630
1975	22,820
1976	25,340
1977	27,980
1978	30,830
1979	33,880
1980	37,110

trends, and what impact they are each likely to have in the future. Careful consideration should be given to analyzing why the historical data moved in the direction it did and what forces could influence future utilization.

The previous example of obstetrical patient days was the actual historical utilization experienced by a 300-bed hospital in the

Figure 4.3

GRAPH OF SECOND DEGREE TREND BY LEAST SQUARE METHOD

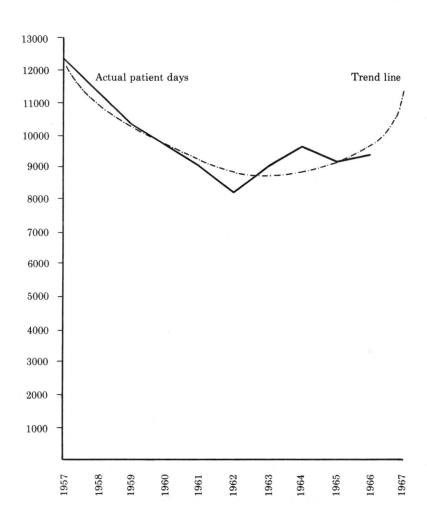

northeast. As shown by the data, hospital officials observed a declining occupancy of obstetrical beds from 1954 into the early 1960s and were determined to do something about it. Convinced that the downward trend was due to the condition of its physical facilities and the decreasing number and increasing age of its obstetricians, the hospital attempted to reverse the trend by a modernization and recruitment program. Early in 1963 a $3 million renovation of the obstetrical floor was completed and, two young obstetricians were appointed to the staff.

Meanwhile, another, smaller hospital several blocks away was also experiencing critically low occupancy levels for obstetrics. But its officials came to a different conclusion about the future. In 1963 this competitive institution closed its obstetrical facilities and converted them to medical-surgical beds. This combination of events caused what appeared to be a dramatic shift in the 300-bed hospital's utilization of obstetrical beds for 1963 and 1964, and hospital officials projected a rosy future as shown in Figure 4.4.

Using a freehand drawing of a trend line between the 1962 and 1964 data points, the hospital's planners projected that obstetrical patient days would return to their former 12,000 level by 1967. Based on this projection these planners were confident of the wisdom of their $3 million capital expenditure and attempted to recruit more obstetricians to the hospital's staff.

Unfortunately, no one associated with this hospital had paid serious attention to the one underlying force that was to have the most significant impact on future utilization of obstetrical facilities: a declining birth rate nationwide. A number of factors are responsible for this birth rate trend. First, the impact of the World War II baby boom was coming to a close. Second, the nation was experiencing changing views toward birth control; and new methods, especially the celebrated "pill" were becoming more readily available. Third, smaller families were becoming more fashionable as world demographers were predicting an uncontrollable population explosion and depletion of the earth's natural resources. In addition to a declining birth rate, modern medical practice was shortening the length of stay for hospitalized mothers.

For our 300-bed hospital, the future use of obstetrical facilities was really not as rosy as hospital officials would have had us

Figure 4.4
GRAPH OF FREEHAND TREND PROJECTION 1957-1964

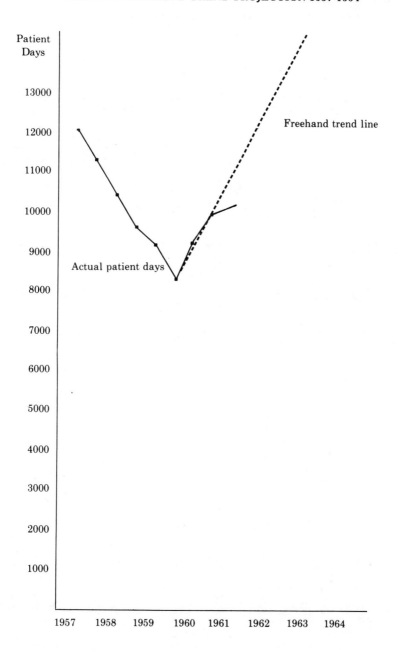

believe. Shown in Figure 4.5 are the actual patient day volumes through 1975, compared with the three trend projections previously demonstrated.

In this case, the linear trend line turned out to be a fairly accurate predictor of future utilization in 1975. But this was so because

Figure 4.5

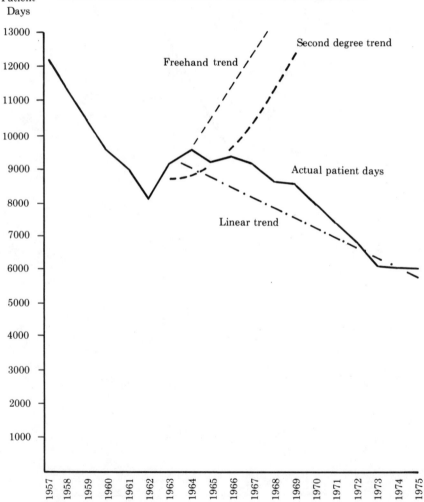

COMPARISON OF ACTUAL OBSTETRICAL PATIENT DAYS WITH TREND LINES CONSTRUCTED UNDER THREE METHODS

the major underlying force in the data (declining birth rate) was moving in a downward linear pattern. The important consideration is that a careful analysis of the underlying causes of historical trends should precede a blind acceptance of a seemingly sophisticated statistical technique.

In projecting future utilization patterns for this hospital from 1975 to 1985, for example, the following questions are among those which need to be addressed:

1. Has the decline the the birth rate leveled off, as might be suggested in the data from 1973-1975?

2. What are the population projections for women of child bearing age (15 to 44)?

3. What are competitive institutions planning, and what has been their utilization experience?

4. What are the trends in average length of stay for mothers?

SUMMARY

Decisions about an institution's future require a sound base of information about the community served and its projected use of health services. The nature of the external environment can be assessed in great detail, and population characteristics can be enumerated endlessly; but both are usually a mistake for most long range planning by health institutions. The most important information about the external environment is that which helps an institution answer some key questions about its future. The exact nature of those questions will, of course, depend on specific circumstances, but there are a few basics that are common to most situations.

1. Which population does an institution serve, and which should it serve?

2. How will the population use your institution's services? Is that use appropriate? Are there unmet community needs?

3. How will changes in community life or services affect population use of your health services?

4. How will decisions by other health institutions affect your institution's planning? Are cooperative arrangements appropriate and feasible?

5. What are the community's objectives and plans as documented in the HSA's Health System Plan? Are your institution's plans consistent, and if not how can the differences be justified?

Most institutions will base their future plans on an analysis of an institution's history and how it arrived at its present situation, coupled with a view of the likely events that will change the past and shape the future. Analyzing the past often necessitates a consideration of the trends in the population's use of an institution's services. But, trend analysis and the conclusions derived therefrom should be used with discriminaton by an institution's planners. Trend analysis can result in misleading conclusions about the future if the techniques and their limitations are not understood. Trend analysis is useful only to the extent that one attempts to understand the underlying causes of historical trends and how forces change and affect future patterns.

Notes

1. Bergwall Reeves, and Woodside, *Introduction to Health Planning* (Washington, D.C.: Information Resources Press, 1974), Chapter 7.
2. William A. Reinke, *Health Planning Qualitative Aspects and Quantitative Techniques* (Baltimore, Md.: Waverly Press, Inc., 1973), pp. 200-201.
3. For source of Demographic Data see Bergwall et al., *Introduction to Health Planning* (Washington, D.C.: Information Resources Press, 1974), pp. 108-115.
4. Primary service area was defined in this case as those geographic areas of the community that account for approximately 80 percent of the hopsital's patient load. A secondary service area was considered to be those geographic locations that accounted for the next 10 percent of the hospital's discharges. The percentages used could vary depending on how the data are grouped.
5. For an excellent bibliography on studies of factors effecting utilization see L. Aday and R. Eichborn, *The Utilization of Health Services, Indices and Correlates* (Washington, D.C.: National Center for Health Services Research and Development, 1972).
6. This subject is discussed from another perspective later in this chapter under "Hazards of Predicting the Future."
7. An excellent examination of the ways to achieve involvement in the community health system is *Guidelines for Hospital Involvement* (Chicago: American Hospital Association, 1973).
8. This method is referred to as least squares. Such a line has two mathematical characteristics. The algebraic sum of the deviations around such a line is zero, and the sum of the squares of the deviations around such a line is a minimum.

Suggested References

American Hospital Association *The Practice of Planning in Health Care Institutions.* Chicago: American Hospital Association, 1973.

Bergwall, David F.; Reeves, Philip N.; and Woodside, Nina B. *Introduction to Health Planning.* Washington, D.C.: Information Resources Press, 1974.

Donabedian, A. "Assessment of Need." *Aspects of Medical Care Administration: Specifying Requirements for Health Care.* Cambridge, Mass.: Harvard University Press, 1973. Chapter 3.

Drosness, D. et al. "The Application of Computer Graphics to Patient Origin Study Techniques." *Public Health Reports* 80, no. 1 (Jan. 1965): 33-40.

Griffith, John. *Quantitative Techniques for Hospital Planning and Control.* Lexington, Mass.: Lexington Books, 1972.

Lubin, Jerome W. et al. "Highway Network Minimum Path Selection Applied to Health Facility Planning." *Public Health Reports* 80, no. 9 (Sept. 1965): 771-778.

Meade, James. "A Mathematical Model for Deriving Hospital Service Areas." *International Journal of Health Services* 4, no. 2 (Spring 1974): 353-364.

Reinke, William A. *Health Planning Qualitative Aspects and Quantitative Techniques.* Baltimore, Md.: Waverly Press, Inc., 1973.

Sigmond, Robert M. "Hospital Discharge Abstract Systems and Institutional Planning." *Medical Care* VIII, no. 4 (July-August 1970): 169-174.

Chapter 5

Analyzing the Internal Environment

In assessing the internal environment for planning, the planning committee of an institution should be concerned primarily with whether the existing organization and facilities will be prepared to respond to a changing external environment. The major factors to be examined internally can be grouped into the following three categories:

1. appraisal of physical facilities,
2. appraisal of manpower availability and composition, and
3. appraisal of financial position.

PHYSICAL FACILITIES

The services of an institution and the manpower that provides those services function through the utilization of physical *spaces,* so *designed* to support specific *functions*. Most health facility obsolescence derives from qualitative or quantitative changes in facility functions and the resulting shortage or inadequate configuration of existing spaces. An examination of each functional space allocation is, therefore, a first step in appraising the state of physical facilities.

Evaluation of space implies the use of standards or norms by which nonconforming variances can be identified. How does one evaluate, for example, how much more space is required for a given laboratory to operate efficiently, given an existing or projected volume of services? How does one judge the capacity of an existing facility to respond to projected changes in patient demand?

It is not possible to develop a single set of space standards against which all existing health facilities can be measured. Space requirements derive from combinations of such factors as demand generated by inpatients as well as ambulatory care, by the teaching responsibilities of an institution, by the medical staff's interests, and by the institution's role in the community. The variations in program among institutions of even the same size are so great that no single standard of space requirements can be uniformly applied. Various guidelines concerning these space allocations, utilized by hospital consultants and architects, have been derived from experience with the design and construction of a wide range of health facilities. Earlier applications of these standards judged all space requirements by the allocation of gross floor area per bed. While this measure still serves as a good estimate of space need for some departmental services, other space requirements are more directly related to workload, such as number of procedures or examinations produced.

One of the most recently reported guidelines on space criteria were developed by the Hospital Survey Committee of the Philadelphia-South Jersey Metropolitan Area following a nationwide study of 65 hospitals over 150 beds built between 1961 and 1967. Displayed in Tables 5.1 and 5.2 are the guidelines generated by this study.[1]

Table 5.1

RECOMMENDED CRITERIA RELATING SPACE TO WORKLOAD, BY SERVICE

		Ratios		
Service	Lower	Median	Upper	Measurement
Laboratories	46.88	51.88	56.88	Procedures per square foot
Diagnostic radiology	4.10	4.35	4.60	Procedures per square foot
Surgery	0.56	0.69	0.82	Procedures per square foot
Food preparation	54.00	61.50	69.00	Meals prepared per square foot
Cafeteria	32.50	35.75	39.00	Meals served per square foot
Emergency	6.25	6.60	6.95	Visits per square foot

Reprinted with permission of the Hospital Survey Committee, Phila., Penna.

Table 5.2

SUGGESTED GUIDELINES RELATING SPACE TO WORKLOAD OR HOSPITAL
SIZE

Department	Variable Related to Space Allocation	Mean Ratio of National Hospitals
Outpatient clinics	Workload	3.42 visits per square foot
Inhalation therapy	Total beds	2.04 square feet per bed
Labor and delivery	Total beds	13.66 square feet per bed
Nursery	Total beds	9.83 square feet per bed
Recovery	Workload	4.95 patient hours per square foot
Physical medicine	Total beds	12.36 square feet per bed
Central service	Total beds	7.95 square feet per bed
General stores	Total beds	28.48 square feet per bed

Reprinted with permission of the Hospital Survey Committee, Phila., Penna.

To illustrate how these guidelines can be used to evaluate the capacity of a service department, let's consider the food preparation area of a 300-bed community teaching hospital. The dietary department projects that approximately 418,500 meals will be prepared during the current fiscal year in the present 5,120 square foot space. Assuming a heavy workload for this department due to size and space efficiencies, the upper ratio of 69.00 meals prepared per square foot will be applied as follows:

418,500   69.00   6,065 gross square feet.

The existing space assigned to food preparation is, therefore, only 84 percent of the size required to produce the existing volume of work efficiently if the upper ratio is taken as the criteria. An evaluation of each departmental space in the institution by the above method can produce one picture of facility adequacy and expansion priorities.

But, space is only one measure of facility adequacy. For example, having a sufficient number of operating rooms in the surgical suite does not guarantee the adequacy of the suite. The unit could have been designed in such a way that it cannot be zoned properly or operated efficiently, or its location might not permit desirable relationships with other departments, such as emergency or

Figure 5.1

FUNCTIONAL ANALYSIS OF SPACE RELATIONSHIPS

Instructions:

For each intersection of two departments, place a code number if a functional relationship exists. The first code identifies the reason for this relationsip.

Next, place a code letter indicating the importance of departmental proximity

Code	Closeness
A	Absolutely necessary
I	Important
U	Unimportant
X	Undesirable

Code	Reason
1	Simplify routing instructions
2	Control patient flow
3	Transfer of speciments
4	Doctor effectiveness
5	Patient and escort comfort
6	Nurse effectiveness
7	Source of supply
8	Patient movement
9	Common resources
10	Noise and confusion
11	Administrative control
12	
13	
14	

1	Administration
2	Boiler room
3	Cafeteria
4	Central linen room
5	Central supply
6	Dietary
7	Emergency
8	Employee facilities
9	Formula room
10	Housekeeping office
11	Laboratory
12	Main laundry
13	Maintenance shop
14	Mechanical equipment rooms
15	Medical nursing unit
16	Medical records
17	Medical staff library
18	Medical-Surgical nursing unit
19	Newborn nursery
20	Nursing service offices
21	OB-delivery suite
22	OB-nursing unit
23	Orthopedic clinic
24	Orthopedic nursing unit
25	Pediatric clinic
26	Pediatric nursing unit
27	Pharmacy
28	Physical therapy
29	Radiology
30	Recovery room
31	Sewing room
32	Stores
33	Surgery
34	Surgical nursing unit

radiology. Departments with inappropriate design, operational, or locational features often require considerably more space than a unit more appropriately designed. Further, the life cycle costs associated with an inefficient design or location could threaten the financial solvency of a department or result in increased rates to patients. One medium-sized hospital found that lack of functional continuity between departments providing patient services resulted in $145,000 in annual excess personnel costs associated with the patient transport and delivery system. This excess cost added approximately $2.00 to patient day charges, not to mention the excess corridor traffic and elevator usage.

One relatively easy method for analyzing departmental location and relationships is through the use of a matrix chart that provides a means to evaluate the relationship of each department to all others. Figure 5.1 demonstrates how this method is applied.

Any two departments listed on the chart have a unique space representing their intersection. Each intersection can then be analyzed for a variety of attributes, in this case the importance of their closeness or distance from each other and the rationale for this decision. For example, the intersection marked (x) indicates that it is undesirable for the laboratories and administration offices to be located physically in close proximity. On the other hand, the intersection marked (4A) shows that it is important for the recovery room to be close to the surgical suite for doctor effectiveness. The analysis then proceeds by comparing the ideal relationships with those that actually exist.

A thorough analysis of departmental design and function usually requires the services of a qualified consultant or experienced architect. The kinds of questions that should be raised in this analysis should include, but not necessarily be limited to, the following:

1. Can the work of the department be carried out safely? Are there proper safeguards against known hazards, including life and fire safety considerations?

2. Is the work space of the department in conformity with current codes, ordinances, and regulations governing construction and operation?

3. Can the work of the department be done reasonably efficiently given its size, configuration, layout, arrangement, and location?

4. What is the quality of the work space, including lighting, ventilation, finishes, air conditioning, clinical utilities, plumbing, power, scientific casework, equipment, and furnishings?

Moving beyond an evaluation of each departmental space, the appraisal of physical facilities must consider the plant as an organic whole, not merely a collection of departments or buildings. The way in which the components are related to one another and function together is as important as the quality of individual work spaces. The age of the structures and their juxtaposition on the site should be studied with respect to future growth patterns and priorities. Among the more important questions that should be raised during this phase of the appraisal are

1. What is the capability for individual departments to respond to independent pressure for expansion with minimum disturbances to each other?

2. How developed is the existing site, and what possibilities exist for future land use? How adequate is the size of the property?

3. What is the structural and design quality of existing buildings and their projected technological life?

4. What is the overall quality and rating of building system components including structural construction; egress system; internal and external circulation systems; heating, ventilating, and air conditioning system; electrical system; plumbing and water supply system; and communication system?

MANPOWER AVAILABILITY AND COMPOSITION

Physicians provide patients, and patients keep a health facility in business. Therefore, the continuing availability of a loyal complement of physicians is essential for the long term survival and development of a health institution. Analysis of the external environments could indicate a certain level of population demand for health services, but unless physicians admit those patients to the institution in sufficient numbers that demand is only on paper or in some other facility. Any appraisal of physician availability and composition should include an analysis of the following information about the medical staff:

1. age distribution,
2. specialty composition,
3. patient admissions,
4. institutional affiliations, and
5. office locations.

The above information could be collected from existing records or questionnaires and displayed in a table. The important considerations of each of the above factors are discussed in the following sections.

Age Distribution

The key question here is whether there is and will continue to be a stable complement of physicians through the infusion of a constant stream of young, recent graduates to replace older retiring staff members. The implications of finding an unstable situation with respect to medical staff replenishment are numerous, including the need to institute a physician recruitment program, relocate the facility, make the existing facility more attractive to young physicians, or reexamine population demand for care. Clearly the solution does not automatically surface when the lack of age stability is found, but only after a careful study of the underlying causes of the problem.

After displaying on a chart the age of each active member of the medical staff and the number of years of affiliation with the institution, the certain questions should be asked.

1. What is the average age of the staff, and has that average changed significantly over the past ten years?
2. Are there a large number of doctors close to retirement age, which could create major voids within the next ten years?
3. How many new physicians affiliate with the institution each year, and is this adequate to compensate for natural attrition?

Specialty Composition

In addition to the overall average age of the medical staff concern should be directed at the average age by specialty. Each of the questions stated above needs to be asked for each medical specialty to focus more clearly on specific voids that could exist. For example, physician replenishment might only be a problem with respect to surgeons and the cause of the problem could be a tyrannical chief of service, rather than a factor external to the institution.

Many of the major programs of a health facility depend on an adequate number of certain medical specialties. Long range plans for the expansion of a rehabilitation service, for example, would necessitate a sufficient supply of physicians trained in physical medicine. Failure to maintain the right complement of these doctors could seriously jeopardize the program.

Patient Admissions

Physician affiliation does not guarantee patient admissions of sufficient numbers to support a health facility's programs. Through multiple institutional appointments, physicians make choices of where they wish to admit their patients. The number of admissions by each member of the medical staff is, therefore, a good indicator of physician loyalty and support for an institution's program. Coupled with age and specialty data, patient admissions by physician can reveal some interesting planning information. For example, one might find that a small group of physicians that will be shortly reaching retirement age account for a high portion of admissions. Perhaps a large group of young doctors have not yet developed strong loyalties, as evidenced by their admission of only a small number of patients to an institution. A complete analysis of the latter situation would also require information on all institutional affiliations of physicians and the percent of their hospitalized patients admitted to each institution.

Institutional Affiliations

While often difficult to obtain, information on multiple appointments held by an institution's physicians can provide useful planning data. It becomes particularly important to detect if physician loyalties appear to be shifting away from an institution over time. Information on multiple appointments can be exchanged by cooperating institutions and is often available through community planning bodies. Physicians can be asked to indicate their other hospital affiliations. Number of admissions to each institution is much more difficult to obtain, but well worth the effort. Physicians can also be asked to provide the percentage of their admissions to an institution, but this information, while extremely valuable for institutional planning, is often difficult to obtain.

Office Locations

Where physicians' offices are located to a large extent determines their patient mix and institutional preferences. It is precisely for this reason that a number of hospitals have built office buildings adjacent to inpatient facilities.

A hospital wishing to be recognized as a major health provider to specific populations or communities must have affiliating physicians who have offices in locations that are convenient to those populations. Likewise, physicians can be expected to optimize their time and minimize their travel by utilizing health facilities that are convenient to their offices. Physicians, admission patterns can, therefore, often be understood by an analysis of office locations.

Physician Attitudes

In addition to the analysis of information about the medical staff, it is often helpful to seek their views through questionnaires on a variety of issues relating to the operation or development of an institution. Below is a partial list of questions, in no particular order, that could be supplemented with other information relevant to specific situations.

1. Would you favor the construction of a doctors' office building? Would you consider renting space?
2. Does this institution have adequate beds?

3. Are there any major voids in service you require for your patients?

4. Are there a sufficient number of physicians on the staff in all specialties? If not, which ones are lacking?

5. If you have multiple hospital appointments, what circumstances normally cause you to prefer another institution for admission of your patients?

6. Are the facilities here adequate to practice your specialty?

7. What do you consider the priority developmental needs of the institution?

Other Health Manpower Availability

Although physician availability will play a key role in future planning by a health institution, the need for and availability of registered nurses, practical nurses, aides, laboratory technologists, x-ray technicians, physical therapists, social workers, dieticians, and others will influence the future capability of an institution.

A number of hospitals have found, for example, that irrespective of a high level of demand for its inpatient services, the unavailability of qualified registered nurses has forced closure of badly needed nursing units. One wonders if such units would have been built had someone been able to project that the hospital's management would not be able to staff them with qualified nursing personnel. Among the questions that need to be raised by an institution's planners in appraising the availability of health manpower are the following:

1. How many individuals of each health occupation are presently employed by health institutions in the area, and what budgeted vacancies exist?

2. What training programs exist in each of these occupations, and what are enrollment and graduation trends?

3. What is the level of community retention of graduates—how many remain in the community to practice their professions?

4. Are the institution's salaries and benefits competitive with other community employers or institutions outside the community?

5. Are living and working conditions favorable for attracting sufficient individuals to work in the institution or the community?

6. What new educational programs, incentives, or recuritment efforts are warranted?

FINANCIAL FEASIBILITY

Health facilities engaged in a comprehensive planning process need to have an early indication of their capacity to incur new debt and how their financial position is likely to be evaluated by lending institutions. However, as is so often the case, a hospital board sets a new project budget, engages an architect, and much later—after considerable expenditure and many planning sessions—the board commissions a financial feasibility study to determine if the project can be paid for. A number of institutions have found that as a result of this process they have had to scale the project down to meet recognized debt limits or shore up the institution's financial operations to gain favorable ratings in the bond markets. Current financial position and potential of the health facility is an internal environment constraint that should be evaluated prior to launching major programs. In the long run, such an analysis can prevent unwise capital expenditures.

The parts of such an analysis of financial feasiblity are much the same as those covered in the more formal studies normally carried out prior to capital financing. The study should include at least the following:

1. historical financial statements and statistics for at least five years, presented to show hospital ability to meet financial obligations; and

2. details of reimbursement mix and contracts sufficient to indicate past and present ability to meet financial obligations from patient care revenue.[2]

Armed with this kind of information on the financial position of the institution, the planning committee can test out the implications of various project costs and make more intelligent decisions on short and long range programs. The committee will know where the institution stands with respect to borrowing capacity and hospital endowments.

SUMMARY

Once the nature of the external environment for planning is understood and projections are made of future utilization patterns, the key question that emerges is whether existing institutional facilities and resources will be able to respond accordingly. The major factors to be examined in such an analysis are the adequacy of physical facilities, manpower availability and composition, and the institution's financial position.

Physical facilities are commonly evaluated, first, from the standpoint of existing space allocations. Applying recognized standards and norms, this analysis provides a "first cut" in judging if spaces are adequately sized for present and future utilization levels. But space is only one measure of facility adequacy. The design and function of departmental spaces and their relationship to each other affect facility obsolescence and life cycle costs. An analysis of the existing site and the quality and distribution of facilities thereon provides important information on future land use and expansion potential.

Equally important, there must be a loyal complement of physicians keeping those facilities occupied. Those physicians not only must be available to the population but also must choose to make an institution their primary affiliation. An analysis of their age distribution, specialty composition, admission patterns, institutional affiliations, and office locations will provide important clues to the likelihood of future physician adequacy. Equally important will be adequate numbers of workers in the other health professions to make it possible for an institution to staff and operate at required levels.

Finally, analysis of an institution's financial position will indicate whether future facility or major program obligations are possible, and what additional resources might be required. This analysis provides a statement of the institution's financial health and capacity to incur further debt—given existing patient demand levels and reimbursement patterns.

Notes

1. Hospital Survey Committee, *Cost Containment and Financing of Hospital Construction* (Philadelphia, Pa.: Hospital Survey Committee, 1974), pp. 9-15.
2. American Hospital Association, *Capital Financing for Hospitals* (Chicago: American Hospital Association, 1974), p. 7.

Suggested References

American Hospital Association. *Capital Financing for Hospitals*. Chicago: American Hospital Association, 1974.

Hospital Survey Committee. *Cost Containment and Financing of Hospital Construction*. Philadelphia, Pa.: Hospital Survey Committee, 1974.

Mille, Alden B., ed. *Functional Planning of General Hospitals*. New York: American Association of Hospital Consultants, McGraw-Hill Company, 1969.

Rosenfield, I. *Hospital Architecture and Beyond*. Reinhold Book Corporation, 1969.

Chapter 6

Developing Mission, Role, and Objectives

WHY REEXAMINE INSTITUTIONAL OBJECTIVES?

Much has been written about the importance of goal development to the institutional planning process. It has only been in recent years that questions have been raised about the nature and structure of health institution objectives. Previously it was generally conceded that there was basically one objective for a health institution, that of "quality patient care." But there is a growing recognition that most institutions have multiple aims and broader social responsibilities. Few would disagree with the notion that all organizations need a purpose for existence toward which their energies and resources can be committed. Clearly, institutional objectives, if clearly delineated and followed, should focus the direction of institutional programs and provide a benchmark to evaluate achievement.

The provision of quality patient care along with research and education are the objectives most often stated by hospital officials. Certainly most observers would seriously question whether a health facility should stay in business if it did not provide quality patient care. But the historical objectives of health institutions are being challenged by many observers of the health care scene as being insufficient, and health care executives are being told to review institutional objectives critically and redirect some of the major efforts of their organizations.

In its *Planning Guide for Hospital Long Range Plans* the New Jersey State Health Planning Council recommends that the following questions should be carefully considered by decision makers in evaluating the mission of an institution:

What population does the institution serve? What are its present characteristics? What are its most important health needs? Are these needs being met by existing institutions and agencies? How well are they being met?

Are there any groups within this population whose health needs are not being met or who are underserved? If this is so, what are the reasons? What efforts should the institution make in this regard?

Is the present mission of the institution relevant to the present needs of the population it serves? What do the institution's various publics think of it and its service? What are the specific patient care services provided by the institution? What is the quality of each of these services? What is the volume of each service? Is the volume sufficient to achieve reasonable economies of scale? Are these programs essential to the present mission of the institution? Do they duplicate the services of neighboring institutions?

What is the role of the institution in the health care system of the area? How do the institution's existing programs and services fit into the overall health care system? What levels of health care does it provide? What arrangements exist to assure that patients requiring services not available in its own facility are referred to other organizations in the area where such services are available?

What is the quality of the institution's overall program? Does it meet or exceed generally accepted standards of the local community? of the area? of the region? of the nation?

Would the institution's patient clientele be better served if any of these services were integrated or combined with the program of another institution? Should any of these programs be dropped because of low volume, poor quality, inadequate resources or irrelevancy?

What are the scope and quality of the institution's ambulatory care services? Do they meet the needs and expectations of local residents?

Does the institution operate or use an emergency ambulance service? Is the service properly staffed with trained personnel? Is the emergency room capable of providing a satisfactory range of emergency services?

Are services provided or have arrangements been made for the care of long-term patients? drug abusers? alcoholics? the mentally ill? Is the institution willing to accept the challenge of caring for such patients if such programs seem indicated in its neighborhood or local community?

What are the educational commitments of the institution? What changes are necessary or desirable to improve them?

What educational arrangements or affiliations does the institution have with medical schools? Is the affiliation meaningful to both institutions?

What are the institution's research capabilities? Are its present research activities an important part of the institution's overall programs? Is sufficient space available for this activity?

What is the nature and extent of the institution's commitments to non-staff physicians in its neighborhood or local community?

Is the Board of Trustees supportive of the administrative leadership of the institution? Is the Board representative of the community served by the institution? What steps has it taken in recent years to seek community input and attitudes to guide in its deliberations?

Is the medical staff organized and qualified? What is the average age of the staff? Have new members been added in recent years? Is there a fulltime staff? How are they selected? What are their responsibilities? What is their contribution to the overall effectiveness of the institution?

Does the institution encounter any unusual difficulties in recruiting and retaining personnel?

Are the institution's financial resources and income

capable of supporting its various programs and commitments in accordance with desired standards?

How does the future promise to affect these programs and commitments? Are there any anticipated external happenings which will change what the institution is doing or presently not doing? How will such events or trends affect the capability of the institution to carry out its mission or its programs? Is the institution willing to commit itself to offer new services, to extend it present services, or to reach new population groups? Is the institution prepared to make the necessary changes in structure, programs, or facilities? What "business" will the institution be engaged in five years from now? ten years from now? [1]

When thoughtful hospital officials have attempted to reexamine institutional objectives, the process has often resulted in time-consuming months of endless board meetings, heated debates, and the painful questioning of strongly held beliefs and values. Under this kind of difficult environment some institutions have found that they can't move the planning process beyond "first base." But, given today's health planning requirements, hospitals and other health facilities must find ways to get beyond the debate and seek resolution on organizational objectives that complement community health objectives. Then, institutions must demonstrate by programs and actions that they have developed more than "paper objectives" for public consumption and that they are committing sufficient resources to achieving expected results. Following is an example of how one hospital went about this process.

A CASE STUDY ON DEVELOPING HOSPITAL OBJECTIVES

Memorial Hospital was established in 1897. For the past seventy-six years the hospital had been maintained as a vital force for the well being of the people of Fairview County. The scope and quality of its services had kept pace with its expanding volume of patient care, and it maintained full accreditation by the Joint Commission on the Accreditation of Hospitals.

The role of this hospital from its inception was that of a community general acute hospital, which provided the basic care services of medicine, surgery, obstetrics and pediatrics, along with formally organized outpatient clinics. Throughout the course of its history the city of Fairview and Memorial Hospital in particular had enjoyed the reputation of being the focal point for hospital and health care activities for the entire upper half of the state.

In the early 1970s the hospital was facing a number of complex issues that were forcing a comprehensive evaluation of its present and future. By tradition, Memorial Hospital had always been recognized as the leader in medical care in the entire upper state. The excellent medical staff had been built up around this premise. In recent years, however, the hospital seemed to have lost some of the prestige and reputation it once enjoyed.

The volume of patient services in many of the departments declined. There was a critical shortage of space, and there were elements of the physical plant that were in need of modernization. There was a distinct awareness among some members of the governing board that the hospital perhaps had not achieved through its organization and operation an optimum degree of effectiveness. In 1970 the hospital was turned down on its application for federal Hill-Burton funds to support plans for new construction because requirements for planning had not been met.

The administrator of Memorial Hospital had held the position since 1970. He was hired shortly after Memorial Hospital's application for federal funds was rejected because of the lack of a long range plan of development. On assuming his position, one of the early tasks he undertook was to analyze the hospital and its potential. He recognized that any future expansion or modernization would have to be based on a sound planning process, and he recognized that a planning process must evolve from the history and precedents of an institution, that he must be sensitive to the attitudes and opinions of key individuals. From the corporate charter creating the institution in 1897 he found that, as originally conceived, *"The purpose of this organization is to provide hospital care to the community."* After reviewing past minutes of the Board of Trustees and policy statements, he found that the institution had not reexamined its role, mission, or goals since 1897.

The administrator knew that if Memorial Hospital were to continue to survive and grow in its service to the community, it would have to examine its role and goals continuously and be prepared to meet the changing needs of the community it serves. He was well aware that society's health needs and expectations are changing and that the area served by Memorial Hospital appeared to be changing.

During the early months following his appointment he held a number of private meetings with individual members of the board and medical staff to begin to develop important relationships, and at the same time assess attitudes and aspirations about the future role and goals of the hospital. From his conversations, he began to compile a lengthy list of different mission statements each of which had various implications for the future direction of the institution and its programs of service. Following are those statements from his notes. Notice that while some of these goals are complimentary, others are in conflict.

1. To provide high quality patient care at a price the community can afford.

2. To insure by efficiency of operation the effective utilization of facilities and services to maintain the fiscal solvency of the institution.

3. To insure excellence by the scope and quality of our services and programs that we maintain and improve our role as a major health center.

4. To keep pace with medical technology and changing concepts of medical practice so our institution can excel in its performance as the central health care resource in this community.

5. To serve as the major referral center in this region for specialized medical services.

6. To provide one class medical service for all patients regardless of their source of payment.

7. To provide comprehensive health services to the community.

8. To provide quality patient services in a way which considers the safety, dignity, and privacy of patients.

9. To provide health services consistent with the expressed needs of the people in this community.

10. To improve the health of the community.

The Planning Committee of the board, which had been created prior to the appointment of the present administrator, began deliberating on the future mission, role, and goals of the institution. With the help of an outside consultant they critically examined both the external environment and internal constraints for planning. And, they spent many long and difficult evenings debating the future role of the institution. At one point in the process a serious impass was reached when the medical staff and the board disagreed on the inclusion of a single sentence in a new mission statement. Compromise was finally achieved through the efforts of a skilled and dedicated committee chairman, who got the committee to endorse a number of resolutions that confirmed areas of agreement and served as a constructive building block for future decisions. The following resolutions were approved:

> That Memorial Hospital faces serious threats to the survival of its programs and services as presently constituted, unless constructive actions are taken to address changing community and institutional needs.

> That in order to obtain favorable community support for future programs, a hospital mission and role statement should be developed which reflects consideration for published community health goals.

> That a plan of development should be designed and implemented which carries out the mission, role and goals of the institution.

The strength of the above resolutions is that they provided the committee chairman an opportunity to build on agreement and overcome stumbling blocks by focusing on committee purpose and objectives. As might be suspected, the process didn't entirely eliminate controversy; but it did help to achieve compromise on the following statement of mission and role.

Example of a Mission and Role Statement

After six months of meetings the planning committee of Memorial Hospital agreed to recommend a mission and role statement for board approval. The following statement came after often heated debate, conflict, and compromise. Even after agreement was reached, some members of the committee were pessimistic that the stated role could ever be implemented by the institution. The committee found that because these statements met with varying interpretation, clarifying paragraphs were helpful in solidifying agreement, as shown below.

MISSION

The mission of the institution is, (1) to function as a leading but integrated component in Fairview County's health care system; (2) to function as the major referral center in the upper state health care system; and (3) to function as a catalytic force in upgrading the level of health in the community supported through emphasis on health maintenance, education, and rehabilitation as well as diagnosis and treatment.

ROLE

Memorial Hospital's role in the health care delivery system of Fairview County and the upper state region is expressed by the composite of the following role statements.

Role (1): To act as a responsible provider of high quality planned, nonduplicative general inpatient care to the residents of Fairview County and the nearby areas of surrounding counties.

Planning Committee's Interpretation: Memorial Hospital shall provide general acute inpatient services to the citizens of Fairview and surrounding counties. Such services shall include diagnosis, treatment, patient education, and rehabilitation programs. The undesirability of unnecessary duplication of services within the community is recognized, and thus services will be designed to meet documented need and/or demand and be complementary to existing services. The provision of such services shall be accomplished by joint planning and cooperative efforts with other inpatient facilities of the region where possible and appropriate.

Role (2): To act as a provider of specialized care to the residents of the upper state region by functioning as the referral center in the health care delivery system.

Planning Committee's Interpretation: The necessity for a coordinated regional health delivery system is recognized. Such system should include, among other things, a source of specialized inpatient and ambulatory care to which patients can be referred for care that is not available at the primary inpatient and outpatient level. Memorial Hospital shall function as such a referral center through continued development of appropriate facilities and programs and its specialized medical staff. Coordination will be facilitated through establishing referral patterns from other hospitals and health care providers in the region. Where Memorial Hospital is not able to provide the requisite care because of lack of facilities, programs, or physicians, patterns of referral will be established with other appropriate referral centers. Specialized inpatient and outpatient services provided will be limited to those for which a need and/or demand exists within the upper state region.

Role (3): To supplement the primary ambulatory care available to residents of Fairview County and nearby areas from other providers.

Planning Committee's Interpretation: Memorial Hospital's primary ambulatory care program shall be designed to supplement rather than preempt primary care provided by physicians and other sources. The primary care physician's role as an integrator and coordinator of various components of the health care team is recognized. The advantages of a continuum of ambulatory and inpatient care with common or integrated components is also recognized. Memorial Hospital's primary ambulatory care program shall, therefore, be designed to provide services that can be utilized by primary care physicians in the treatment of their patients and to provide total primary ambulatory care to those population segments that have primary care demands not met by physician-providers.

Role (4): To act as a leading force as well as active participant in the development of effective planning mechanisms for the delivery of health care services to the residents of Fairview County and the upper state region.

Planning Committee's Interpretation: If health care delivery is to be accomplished without unnecessary duplication of and unwarranted gaps in service, the establishment of effective mechanisms for achieving coordination between providers is essential. Memorial Hospital recognizes this fact and feels a commitment to stimulate the development of planning activities as well as participate in those activities. Such planning should include both institutional and other providers of health services. It should be based on realistic needs and demands for health services and incorporate consumer input.

Role (5):   To act as a stimulus in upgrading the level of health in the upper state region through active support of and participation in programs of education and nealth maintence.

Planning Committee's Interpretation: Attainment of high levels of health requires that the provision of services be responsive to existent conditions. The need for education programs for both providers and consumers is recognized. Moreover, the need to establish programs aimed at the prevention of illness, disease, and injury is apparent. Each of these areas requires a multidimensional approach for the attainment of lasting progress. Thus in each, Memorial Hospital recognizes the applicability of established principles and the necessity that it participate along with other individuals, institutions, and agencies in the development and operation of sound programs.

LINKING OBJECTIVES TO INSTITUTIONAL MISSION

A health institution's mission, role, and objectives are not worth much unless human and other resources can be committed to their attainment through operating departments.

Competent health care executives have known for a long time that superior performance requires that each job be directed toward the objectives of the organization and that results should be measured by the contribution they make to the success of the institution. It is, therefore, axiomatic that the more we find each subunit in an organization working toward common organizational objectives in a coordinated way, the more effective that organization is likely to be in achieving its ends.

Within the framework presented here, an objective refers to a desired or needed result to be achieved in some specified long range period.[2] Objectives can be written for every component of the institution that is important enough to have plans. The principal method for developing long range objectives is through the planning process described in this book. It involves the interaction of many people in the development of statements that reflect what they plan to achieve to carry out the mission of the organization.

Linking objectives to the mission of an organization is a time-consuming and imprecise process. It is not always easy to see the connection between the two, and some employees find it difficult to think in terms of contribution to the overall purpose of the organization. However, the links between mission, long range objectives, and short range objectives must be established if the institution is to implement programs and actions with desired results.

One way of looking at the way objectives interlace is demonstrated in Figure 6.1. When conceptually viewed in terms of the model presented, the hospital's mission clearly becomes the overriding direction for all other objectives and actions. Long range objectives (usually five to ten years) should be the next component of the model, for they are the most general and overriding statements of how the hospital plans to carry out its mission in the long run.

A specific set of short range objectives are then stated, which implement each of the long range objectives. Although short range objectives have a greater degree of specificity than long range objectives, they do not state exactly how they will be carried out. Implementation of short range objectives is left for the next level of goal development, namely the operating departments.

RELATING DEPARTMENTAL OBJECTIVES TO INSTITU-
TIONAL OBJECTIVES

Clearly, a health institution achieves its mission and objectives through the work accomplished by its operating departments. It is essential, therefore, that each department head establish departmental objectives consistent with institutional objectives and be encouraged to push the process down into the organization.

One of the most common errors made by health institutions is to stop the linking process at the level of institutional objectives. Department heads are given a published list of company objectives and asked to submit a list of departmental objectives without demonstrating the links. After the fact analysis by management often finds that some departmental objectives are not desirable, or even worse, that some institutional objectives are not being implemented by operating departments. Knowledge of the relationship between departmental objectives and institutional objectives is also essential to management when it attempts to assess departmental accomplishments and contributions.

The following "Objective Responsibility Chart" (Table 6.1) pro-

Figure 6.1

LINKING OBJECTIVES TO MISSION—A MODEL

BASIC MISSION:
To provide or arrange for high quality comprehensive health care services for the population we serve with the goal of improving the health and well-being of that population, within the limits of available resources

Long Range Objectives (5-10 years)

I.	II.	III.	IV.
Develop the diagnostic and treatment services with special emphasis on early detection, rehabilitation and follow-up.	Develop a comprehensive ambulatory care program, emphasis on preventive and extended care, and increased accessibility.	Improve utilization and productivity of present facilities.	Develop manpower resources with emphasis on physician extenders.

Short Range Objectives (1 Year)
(III: UTILIZATION AND PRODUCTIVITY)

1. Strenghten the planning and coordination between services
2. Expand and improve our utilization review program
3. Initiate a management engineering study of a major service
4. Establish mechanisms for measuring productivity.

Table 6.1

OBJECTIVE RESPONSIBILITY CHART

Short Range Objective III-1: *Strengthen the planning and coordination between services.*

To be implemented by these departments as follows:		Target Date	Completed
Transport Department:	Correct inefficiencies in the patient transport system, demonstrating a 10 percent reduction in "down time" without sacrificing quality.	7/ 1	
Business Office and Nursing:	Eliminate missed charges for items dispensed by nursing service	8/ 1	
Purchasing:	Implement an interdepartmental materials management system	6/ 1	
Admission:	Implement an improved bed control system	8/ 30	

vides a convenient way to link objectives and to evaluate accomplishments. Beginning with one of the institution's short range objectives, the chart delineates the responsibilities of each affected department, including the expected date of project completion.

One hospital located in the southeast uses the following cycle to guide its department heads in the development of program objectives:

June and July: Department heads meet with superiors and review planning program, concept of mission and objectives, the development of departmental objectives.

July and August: Department heads meet with supervisors, develop departmental objectives in written form, backed up by narrative description of program, based on planning objectives for the next budget year.

September: Department and administration hold conferences and agree on objectives and narrative description of program for the next budget year. They prepare overall hospital objectives and narrative description of hospital program for the next budget year.

September-October: Overall hospital objectives and program are prepared along with departmental objectives and program description and presented to the board for approval.

October: Approved objectives and program descriptions are shared with department heads, and budget drafts are prepared. Budgets, based on objectives and program descriptions are prepared in detail in prescribed, uniform format, including staffing patterns, salary levels, alterations in space, programmed capital expenditures, etc.

At this same time, the department head prepares program objectives and descriptions for the second and third fiscal year for purposes of Section 234 capital expenditures budgeting. The capital expenditures budget for the two additional fiscal years are prepared in draft form at this time. The additional two years are more in the form of "projections" rather than specific operational instruments. The degree of specificity decreases as time extends into the future.

October: Administration prepares overall budget and program descriptions for next fiscal year for presentation to planning committee and board.

November: Planning committee reviews budget, program descriptions, and objectives for next fiscal year and makes recommendations to the board for approval, either as presented or in modified form. Board considers recommendations, reviews budget, program descriptions and objectives and takes formal action for approval.

December: Approved budget, program descriptions, and objectives are distributed to all operating department heads and become operational as of December 31 for the next fiscal year.

Quarterly intervals during budget year: Progress reports including comparative budget statements are prepared and submitted to operational department heads and the board. Variance from program and budget are responded to by department heads and reported to the board. Formal adjustments in program and operating budgets are prepared as numbered revisions and approved by the board as circumstances require.[3]

What Makes a Good Objective?

Structures of objectives are as varied as structures of health care facilities. Larger institutions usually have a need for the development of objectives in more areas than do smaller ones and could require a more complex framework of linkages. Objectives can be expressed either quantitatively or qualitatively and can include a wide degree of specificity and different time dimensions.

The literature on management by objectives is extensive and will not be repeated here. There are, however, several criteria on what makes a good objective that deserve discussion within the context of the institutional planning function.

The first criteria has to do with responsibility. Perhaps the first test of whether an objective will be accomplished is if the individual responsible for achieving the desired results understands and accepts the objective statement. In an earlier discussion of creating an organizational climate, importance was attached to the creation of a climate which will develop the attitudes, perspectives, and personal commitment to make the implementation of plans feasible. One of the most effective ways to achieve this climate is by permitting employees to participate in the development of those objectives for which they will be held responsible, or for which their actions are expected to make a contribution. Those responsible for carrying out objectives should feel that they are attainable, given the time and resources available.

The second criteria has to do with the achievement of results. Objectives should be as concrete as possible and should state the results to be achieved. In other words, what outcome or behavior is anticipated as a result of the successful accomplishment of the objective? Related to this criteria is the need to specify by what measures one will be able to determine if the objective has been accomplished.

The final criteria involves the importance of delineating the time frame in which the objective is to be accomplished. Time constraints help establish work priorities and enforce accountability. When several individuals or departments are responsible for different objectives, which must be linked at some predetermined time, accountability for meeting completion deadlines can be essential.

SUMMARY

The examination of an institution's mission, role, and objectives is often a difficult, time-consuming, and sometimes painful process. The process could point to suggested changes in philosophy or could open up considerations of major changes in goals or programs. This is the area where resistance to change becomes most clearly manifest and where preparing the right climate for planning is, therefore, essential.

But the difficulties enumerated cannot be used as an excuse to forego the process. The historical objectives of health institutions are being challenged, and those responsible for reviewing and approving institutional plans are evaluating the stated objectives of institutions, and the manner in which those objectives are implemented. The governing body of a health institution will find it a fact of life in future planning that the institution's mission and role in the community will have to be justified in terms of how they implement community health goals.

Recognizing that words come easier than actions, the manner in which an institution implements its pronounced mission and role will be the critical measure of future planning effectiveness. However, the program and services of a health institution are carried out by its operating departments. Therefore, links between the overall mission and role and the long and short range objectives of operating departments must be established if the institution is to implement programs and actions with desired results.

___

Notes

1. N.J. State Health Planning Council, *Planning Guide for Hospital Long Range Plans* (March 21, 1975). (The original version of this list appeared in Joseph P. Peters, *Concept, Commitment, Action* (New York: United Hospital Fund of New York and the Health and Hospital Planning Council of Southern New York, Inc., 1974).

2. There is considerable confusion in the literature on the definition and use of objectives and goals. The two concepts are used interchangeably throughout the planning literature.
3. Vernon D. Seifert, "A Model For Institutional Planning" presented at a seminar on Institutional Planning, Tulane University, November 7-9, 1975.

Suggested References

American Hospital Association. *Guidelines for Hospital Involvement.* Chicago: American Hospital Association, 1973.

American Hospital Association. *The Practice of Planning in Health Care Institutions.* Chicago: American Hospital Association, 1973.

American Hospital Association. *Statement on Planning.* Chicago: American Hospital Association, 1973. pp. 83-86.

Bair, John A. "Long-Range Health Care Planning: A Look at Business Practice Discloses Techniques for Projecting Goals." *Trustee* 22 (August 1969): 23-29.

Hughs, Charles L. *Goal Setting: Key to Individual and Organizational Effectiveness.* New York: American Management Association, 1965.

Chapter 7

Selecting and Using Hospital Consultants

WHEN DO YOU NEED A CONSULTANT?

Health institutions have available to them a wide range of consulting services to help them in decision making. Typically, a consultant is hired when a health facility is contemplating expansion, modernization, or replacement. Consultants, however, are often used for other varied problems, such as when the management staff of an institution does not possess the technical expertise to solve a specific problem. Consultants are also utilized when an organization lacks the necessary experience in the development or implementation of a new program (e.g., an HMO). Frequently, administrators who are unable to convince top management of the correctness of their position on an issue use consultants to sell their viewpoint. Sometimes consultants are used as outside experts to help stimulate management and employees with new concepts in a particular field.

The areas of service provided by hospital consultants today are only limited by the financial resources available for their engagement. Some of the more commonly advertised services are

1. local and regional community surveys;
2. facility role studies and long range planning;
3. hospital programming and assistance in the process of planning, construction, and equipment selection;
4. management and organization evaluation;
5. medical staff organization and relationships;
6. medical care appraisal or audit programs;
7. facility mergers or shared services;

8. financial feasibility studies; and

9. financial planning and capital fund acquisition.

Yet, despite the growing utilization of hospital consultants, many chief executives do not know how to use consultants appropriately. Many know little about consultants, how to select them, work with them, and obtain maximum benefit from their use.

SELECTION PROCESS

The hospital administrator and his governing body are faced with the problem of selecting from a wide array of consultants with varying skills and competencies. To minimize the risk to the organization in receiving poor or inappropriate consultation, careful attention should be given to the selection process. Advice on the selection process can be reduced to six basic principles.

Top management should clearly identify the institutional problem and define its parameters.

Frequently, consultants engaged by an organization are faced with an inadequate definition of the problem to be solved. Clear problem definition is essential to evaluate the problem-solving methodologies of competing bidders for a job. Leaving the parameters of the problem open for interpretation increases the risk of inappropriate or incomplete consultation. Working with his top management staff and the governing body, the chief executive should develop a written understanding of the background data of the problem, the specific problem parameters, and the specific objectives of the consultation. There should be general agreement among these participants that a consultant should be hired to solve the problem or problems. Agreement for his employment is an essential first step, for the consultant, to be effective, must achieve acceptance and credibility by the people in the organization.

Use a variety of sources such as colleagues, former consultants, professional associations, and professional publications to derive potential names of consultants.

It is estimated that in the United States there are 2,700 consulting firms employing over 25,000 professional staff members, as well as 30,000 individuals providing consulting services to government and industry.[1]

A number of the more well-known consulting firms and individuals who have specialized in health facility consultation are members of professional consulting associations. These associations can provide a prospective client with a list of their membership, their qualifications, and affiliations.[2] However, a large number of other firms and individuals provide consulting services to health institutions. Every year a number of individuals splinter off large consulting firms to form their own organizations. In this latter case, the individual and his qualifications become even more important than the name of the firm, which might be little known. A large number of university professors also provide specialized consulting services to institutions and governmental agencies. With this wide array of possibilities, the chief executive officer and his board would be well advised to consider all the options within the framework of an institution's needs before making a selection.

Obtain additional information on potential consultants including background, education, experiences, and publications.

A potential consultant should be expected to provide any information concerning his qualifications that an institution deems necessary in the evaluation process. Information that should be readily available includes:

1. the kinds of services provided,
2. the staff expertise and data support available to his firm (especially important for independent individual consultants), and
3. the previous clients served and the nature of the service.

Check with previous clients to find out about the consultant's past performance.

One of the most valuable elements of the selection process can be the advice of those who have used a consultant's services. That process could also include an on-site visit of any physical structures, programs, or systems resulting from the consultant's recommendations. Information that could be valuable for evaluation includes:

1. the smoothness of working relationships between the client and the consultant,

2. skill demonstrated by the consultant in analyzing the problem,

3. pragmatism of the consultant's recommendations,

4. support or follow-up provided by the consultant during implementation, and

5. accomplishment of the project within the original cost and time estimates.

The individuals who will be working most closely with the consultant should be involved in the selection process.

Hospitals vary considerably in their processes of consultant selection. It is important, however (as in problem definition), for all key members of the top management team to be involved in the selection process. One possibility is for top management to establish a set of criteria to evaluate consultant proposals. The delineation of selection criteria not only forces the crystallization of what is important to a specific institution but also results in a more objective evaluation of alternative consultants. Criteria might be developed along the following five areas:

1. approach used in solving the problem,

2. requirements for assistance by personnel of the organization,

3. qualifications and personal characteristics of the consulting staff,

4. project completion time requirements, and

5. costs for providing services.

The above process of evaluation implies the receipt from each potential consultant of a formal proposal, which describes his interpretation of the problem and its parameters, along with a discussion of at least the five areas listed above.

Interview each potential consultant on a face-to-face basis, and have them indicate how they would approach your problem.

During this interview process it is important for management to recognize that the top man in the consulting firm who "sells the job" is not necessarily the individual who will direct the project. If possible, that individual or individuals should be appointed before a final selection is made, and he, too, should be included in the interview process. Among the more relevant questions that should be addressed by top management during the interview are

1. Is the firm and/or the project director experienced in handling such projects?
2. Does he have adequate special knowledge of the job?
3. Can he work effectively with people? Will he gain respectful acceptance by people in the organization with whom he will come into contact?
4. Is he skilled in analyzing and presenting data?
5. Has he the time to meet the institution's requirements?

EXAMPLE OF SPECIFICATIONS FOR PROPOSALS

Unfortunately, consultants sometimes solve the wrong problems or provide the wrong recommendations because of an inadequate definition of the client institution's problem. Perhaps the first and most crucial ingredient to a successful consulting arrangement is an agreement by both client and consultant of the parameters of the problem and any specifications for the work. Following is an example of how one community approached this issue.

Requests for Proposals

Introduction

The purpose of this study shall be to furnish data to be used as a basis for decision making as to the future courses of action that should be taken regarding health care facilities/services to meet the future needs for health care in Walnut County.

Nature Of The Study

The proposal submitted should address the following questions.

Question 1: What is the potential demand for health care in the identified service area in 1975, 1980, 1990, and 2000 to include the

a. demand for hospital care including projected admissions, patient days, and bed needs for medical, surgical, pediatric, and obstetrical specialties,

b. demand for nursing home care including projected admissions, patient days, and bed needs for the categories of custodial, skilled, and intermediate care services,

c. demand for ambulatory care to include projected outpatient visits for primary care, emergency care, and major specialty care.

Question 2: What is an appropriate design for a health services delivery system that will meet the demands identified in Question 1 for hospital, nursing home, and ambulatory care to include identification of needed facilities and services and health manpower requirements.

Related Questions:

1. Number, size, type, services, organization, and location of facilities needed?

2. Projected ancillary services needed?

3. Projected needs for physicians by specialty, including the number that can be supported in full-time practice and needs for visiting specialists from large medical centers?

4. Projected needs for professional nurses, licensed vocational nurses, and other allied health professionals.

Question 3: Given currently available medical facilities, what specific actions should be taken to improve the current health care delivery system to meet the design developed through answering Question 2? (Specify priorities and time frame).

Related Questions:

1. What health care facilities are presently available in Walnut County including type, services, location, and condition of plant and equipment?

2. What health care facilities are presently available in counties that are contiguous to Walnut County including type, services, location, and condition of plant and equipment? (Consider only those identified as in the service area.)

Question 4: Given present medical manpower, what specific actions should be taken with regard to medical manpower to improve current health care delivery and to meet the design through answering Question 2?

Related Questions:

1. What are the health manpower resources presently available in Walnut County and contiguous counties including numbers by profession, specialty/subspecialty, and present location of practice and/or employment?
2. What additional health manpower resources by profession, specialty and subspecialty will be needed to meet the design developed through answering Question 2?

Question 5: Given the specific actions recommended in response to Questions 3 and 4, what feasible alternatives are available in meeting the health care needs of Walnut County with respect to hospital, nursing home, and ambulatory care?

Related Questions:

1. Feasible use, if any, of the existing facilities?
2. Feasibility of merger or affiliation among existing facilities?
3. Assuming need and feasibility, should a new hospital, nursing home, and ambulatory care clinic be located in one facility?

Question 6: Given a demonstrated need, the design of a health delivery system to meet identified needs, and the presentation of available alternatives as a result of this study, what are the recommendations of the consultant with regard to:

1. Health facilities to be constructed and services to be offered that will be financially feasible (financial feasibility from a prospective lenders viewpoint)?
2. Extent to which increases/decreases in costs/utilization would affect financial feasibility?

3. Advantages/disadvantages of the following options:
county build and operate?
county build and operate through management contract?
build and operate as a nongovernmental, not-for-profit institution?
build and operate by private investor?

4. Costs of developing facilities (maximum amount that could be financed through long-term debt)?

5. Sources of capital financing?

6. Extent to which debt service requirements can be met (that is, does projected cash flow assure a debt service ratio of at least 1:7)? Present supportive analysis.

7. What third-party reimbursement programs exist in support of hospital/nursing home care; and, specifically, what is the consultant's assessment of the available agreements including scope of services covered and adequacy of reimbursement as it relates to services rendered.

Study Specifications

The proposal submitted should include, as a minimum, certain specifications.

1. The cost of conducting the study, including a statement as to whether the cost is firm or is an estimate, and a statement as to whether the cost includes travel and other out-of-pocket expenses.

2. The estimated time of delivery of the final report and the estimated dates that interim progress reports will be submitted.

3. The method of payment of the fee for the study.

4. The qualifications of the individual or individuals who will do the field work and those who will have supervisory responsibility.

5. A clear description of any limitations that the consultant will place on any study areas described in these guidelines.

6. The number of copies of the report that will be delivered.

7. The scope of client review that is included in the base price. (State number of trips/hours consultant is willing to spend with

the Advisory Committee, the Board of Supervisors, and/or the Board of Trustees.)

8. A statement of any direct or indirect relationships that might exist between the consultant and any person or group involved or interested in present or proposed medical facilities in Walnut County shall be included.

CONSULTING PROCESS

Once a consultant has been selected, key employees throughout the organization should be informed of the study objectives and be prepared to provide their cooperation and assistance. Though varying with the nature of the problem, the consultant will normally need to collect a great deal of information about those aspects of the organization that relate to the study objectives. He might need access to files and documents to which limited access is ordinarily allowed. He might need to question employees on the location of specific data and the easiest way to retrieve needed information. He could question the reliability of some information and seek to establish mechanisms for ongoing collection and retrieval of current data. In the process, he will try to learn much about the organization and its problems from employees with whom he comes into contact. He will more than likely need to set up formal interviews with key people and group discussions with others. Only through the commitment and willing assistance of employees throughout the organization will maximum benefits from the consultation be obtainable.

At the project's inception, a timetable should be agreed to by both the client institution and the consultant. Barring unforeseen circumstances the project schedule should be maintained and periodically monitored by someone in the client organization. Periodic reports should be presented to the chief executive and his management team as the work of the project progresses, and any deviations from original intent should be communicated by both parties at that time. At these periodic sessions the consultant should report his progress to date and findings to management and learn from their insights and perceptions. Management, on the other hand, should take this opportunity to provide additional information and feedback to the consultant.

To be effective and have maximum assurance of acceptance and implementation by an organization, a consultant's report must be more than nicely bound recommendations by an outside expert. Many consultant's reports do no more than gather dust on the bookshelves of a client organization. The key to acceptance is the participation and involvement in the study by those who will be doing the accepting. A consultant who brings together the key decision makers in an organization, guides them through every step of the project, injecting their ideas, capitalizing on their insights, addressing their criticisms, and attempting to find compromising solutions, is more likely to arrive at a product that can be implemented when he leaves.

The final report should include specific instructions on how to initiate the consultant's recommendations with timetables and projected costs, when appropriate. The consultant's job is really not complete until an organization implements his recommendations. He should therefore make himself available to give follow-up advice as the implementation proceeds and be prepared to make adjustments to the implementation plan if circumstances warrant that such adjustments be made.

STANDARDS OF PROFESSIONAL CONSULTATION

Health Care Executives employing consultants should be aware of the professional practices governing the conduct of individual management consultants, which are recognized and enforced by reputable firms. The widely respected Code of Professional Ethics adopted by the Association of Consulting Management Engineers (ACME) is binding on management consultants whose firms are members of the association. At the close of this chapter this code and the association's companion statement on obligations of Good Practice appear as Exhibits 7.1 and 7.2. Following these exhibits, the American Association of Hospital Consultants Code of Professional Ethics is presented in Exhibit 7.3. Managers of health care institutions, might find these professional expectations helpful when either judging a consultant's qualifications or evaluating the work performed.[3]

SUMMARY

While more health institutions are utilizing a variety of consultants for many different problems organizations face, many know little about consultants: how to select them, work with them, and obtain maximum benefit from their use. To minimize the risk to an institution in receiving poor or inappropriate advice from consultants, top management should pay careful attention to a well-designed selection process. Six basic principles of consultant selection were discussed. They are

1. clearly define the problem parameters,
2. use a variety of sources,
3. investigate the consultant's qualifications,
4. check with previous clients,
5. involve the management team in selection, and
6. interview the project director.

Exhibit 7.1

CODE OF PROFESSIONAL ETHICS

PREAMBLE

The following articles are intended to aid management consultants individually and collectively in maintaining a high level of ethical conduct. They are standards by which a consultant may determine the propriety of his conduct in his relationships with prospective clients, colleagues, members of allied professions, and the public.

These standards have evolved out of the experience of the members since the Association was incorporated in 1933, and are binding on all member firms and the consultants of their staffs.

ARTICLE I

WE BELIEVE that the principal objective of the profession of management consulting is to help owners and managers in commerce, industry, government and nonprofit organizations analyze and solve management and related operating and technical problems. The chief characteristics of the professional management consultant are integrity, objectivity, analytical skill, specialized knowledge, broad experience, and a practical approach to the solution of management problems.

ARTICLE II

WE WILL FURTHER the public interest by contributing through research and competent counsel on management problems to the development and better understanding of the art and science, practice and role of management in the economic and social systems of the free world.

ARTICLE III

WE WILL PUBLICIZE our firm or services only in a manner upholding the dignity of the profession. We will present our qualifications to prospective clients solely in terms of our ability, experience, and reputation. We will not guarantee any specific amount of cost reduction or increase in profits from our efforts, nor will we accept an engagement where the fee is related to any cost reduction that may result.

ARTICLE IV

WE WILL ACCEPT only those engagements we are qualified to undertake and which are in the best interests of clients.

ARTICLE V

WE WILL CHARGE reasonable fees which are commensurate with the nature of the services performed and the responsibility assumed, and which, whenever feasible, have been agreed upon in advance of the engagement. We will not allow any person to practice in our name who is not in our employ. We will neither accept nor pay fees to persons outside our firm for referral of clients. Nor will we accept fees, commissions, or other valuable consideration from individuals or organizations whose equipment, supplies, or services we may recommend in the course of our work with clients.

ARTICLE VI

WE WILL GUARD as confidential all information concerning the business and affairs of clients coming to us in the course of professional engagements.

ARTICLE VII

WE WILL NOT SERVE clients under terms or conditions which tend to interfere with or impair our objectivity, independence, or integrity.

ARTICLE VIII

WE WILL NEGOTIATE for possible work with a client where another firm is currently engaged only when we are assured there is no reason for conflict between the two engagements.

ARTICLE IX

WE WILL SERVE TWO or more competing clients at the same time on problems in a sensitive area only with their knowledge.

ARTICLE X

WE WILL NOT MAKE direct or indirect offers of employment to employees of clients. If we are approached by employees of clients regarding employment in our firm or in that of another client, we will make certain that we have our clients' consent before entering into any negotiations with such employees.

ARTICLE XI

WE WILL MAKE certain that the members of our professional staff, in order to insure their continuing objectivity, shall under no circumstances use a consulting engagement as a means of seeking new employment for themselves.

ARTICLE XII

WE WILL NOT USE data, technical material, procedures, or developments originated by other consulting firms but not released by them for public use, without their written permission.

ARTICLE XIII

WE WILL REVIEW for a client the work of another consulting firm currently employed by him only with the other consultant's knowledge.

ARTICLE XIV

WE WILL NOT MAKE direct or indirect offers of employment to consultants on the staffs of other consulting firms. If we are approached by consultants of other consulting firms regarding employment in our firm or in that of a client, we will handle each situation in a way that will be fair to the consultant and his firm.

ARTICLE XV

WE WILL ADMINISTER the internal and external affairs of our firm in the best interests of the profession at all times.

ARTICLE XVI

WE WILL ENDEAVOR to safeguard clients, the public and ourselves against consultants deficient in moral character or professional competence. We will observe all laws, uphold the honor and dignity of the profession, and accept self-imposed disciplines. We will respect the professional reputation and

practice of other consultants. But we will expose, without
hesitation, illegal or unethical conduct of fellow members of the
profession to the proper ACME authority.

ARTICLE XVII

WE WILL STRIVE continually to improve our knowledge, skills,
and techniques, and will make available to our clients the
benefits of our professional attainments.

Reprinted with permission of ACME

Exhibit 7.2

OBLIGATIONS OF GOOD PRACTICE

In order to promote highest quality of performance in the practice of management consulting, ACME has formulated the
following standards of good practice for the guidance of the
profession. The member firms subscribe to these practices
because they make for equitable and satisfactory client relationships and contribute to success in management consulting.

1. We make it a practice to confer with an organization that is
considering the use of a management consultant, to discuss the
nature and scope of the assistance that may be required and to
explore the benefits that may be attained. This preliminary discussion may be undertaken without obligation to the prospective client.

2. We recommend the engagement of our services only if we
believe that real financial or other benefits will be realized by
the client.

3. We make certain that the client receives a clear statement of
the objectives and scope of the proposed engagement and when
feasible its approximate cost, and cover this in writing by an in-
itial proposal or a letter of confirmation when we accept the
engagement.

4. We endeavor to accomplish our work expeditiously, consistent with professional thoroughness, and without disrupting the
daily operations of the client organization.

5. We believe that the primary purpose of each engagement is
to develop complete and practical solutions for the problems
under study, including a realistic program for putting them into
effect. Our professional staff is available to help implement
them.

6. We discuss in detail with the client any important changes in
the nature, scope, timing, or other aspects of an engagement,
and obtain his understanding and agreement before we take
any action on them.

7. We acquaint client personnel with the principles, methods, and techniques applied, so that the improvements suggested or installed may be properly managed and continued after completion of the engagement.

8. We maintain continuity of understanding and knowledge of client's problems and the work that has been done to solve them by maintaining appropriate files of reports submitted to clients. These are protected against unauthorized access and supported by files of working papers, consultants' log-books, and similar recorded data.

9. We continually evaluate the quality of the work done by our staff to insure insofar as is possible that all of our engagements are conducted in a competent manner.

10. We endeavor to provide opportunity for the professional development of those men who enter the profession, by assisting them to acquire a full understanding of the functions, duties, and responsibilities of management consultants, and to keep up with significant advances in their areas of practice.

11. We endeavor to practice justice, courtesy, and sincerity in our profession. In the conduct of our practice, we strive to maintain a wholly professional attitude toward those we serve, toward those who assist us in our practice, toward our fellow consultants, toward the members of other professions, and the practitioners of allied arts and sciences.

Reprinted with permission of ACME

Exhibit 7.3

The American Association of Hospital Consultants
CODE OF PROFESSIONAL ETHICS

Preamble

The American Association of Hospital Consultants, a non-profit organization of individual member consultants, was incorporated in 1949 as a professional society for the purposes of serving health care providers. The Association is a multidisciplinary resource of consulting practice; offers continuing education programs to members; and provides education opportunities to individuals and groups interested in health care organization and management.

Integrity is the most valuable asset of the consultant. An AAHC member is normally obligated to those who retain his/her services to give at all times the most conscientious services of which he/she is capable. Clients have a right to expect from the consultant member opinions and judgments which are honest, free from motives of personal gain, based on sound application of knowledge and experience, and in the client's best interest. He/she will avoid practice and conduct likely to bring discredit upon himself/herself or professional colleagues.

Members are, by Association eligibility standards, health care consultants who have devoted essentially full-time to the practice of hospital/health services and facilities and facilities consultation for a minimum of five years and who have been found to meet, for each classification, membership standards of competence and character. All applicants certify in writing their acceptance of the AAHC Code of Professional Ethics as their minimum standard of conduct as a consultant.

Relationship of the Consultant to the Client

1. The AAHC Consultant shall consider service to the client as the primary objective. To this end, the consultant should place the interest of the client ahead of his/her own and serve with competence and integrity.

2. The AAHC Consultant should be impartial in judgments and prevent personal bias and prejudice from influencing decisions which must be based upon an ethically sound objective approach.

3. Confidentiality of client information gathered during a professional assignment shall be maintained and information released only to appropriate individuals or groups with client knowledge and approval.

4. The AAHC Consultant shall make every effort to avoid any potential conflict of interest by informing the client of all relationships, circumstances or interests that might influence the objectivity of judgments and recommendations rendered the client.

5. The AAHC Consultant should be qualified in the area(s) of expertise required, as should any associate assigned to the project. If, during the course of the study or service, other expertise is required—beyond the capability of the individual consultant or his/her firm—the consultant shall make such need known to the client.

6. The AAHC Consultant should not hesitate to disagree with the employing body if in his/her judgment that body is favoring or committing an erroneous conclusion or course of action.

Relationship to Other Consultants/Professionals

7. The relationship of consultants to one another shall always be one of courtesy, professional respect and cooperation. Although opinion may differ respecting the desirability or feasibility of certain proposals or recommendations, these differences of opinion should never lead to written or oral statements or actions not consistent with the professional status and dignity of a consultant. This principle does not imply that he/she should protect a colleague who is obviously guilty of unfair or unethical practices.

8. Consistent with the principle above (5) the consultant should recognize other client-retained professionals as qualified individuals whose skill and knowledge may be in fields parallel, complementary or separate to his/her own.

9. An AAHC member shall accept a client assignment while another consultant is serving that client only after satisfying himself/herself that no conflicts between assignments will exist. A member will agree to replace another professional on the same project only after being ap-

proached by the client and receiving positive assurance that the former consultant has been terminated.

10. When two or more individuals or firms are being considered for the same project, the consultant will not endeavor to improve his/her own position by disparaging the ability of a competitor or by questioning his/her integrity; will not resort to bargaining to undercut competitors, nor endeavor to supplant a competitor in a particular assignment after becoming aware that definite steps have been taken to employ the competitor.

11. A member should encourage and be receptive to cooperative actions between consultants working in the same community or region when such actions can minimize project effort and/or maximize project results; are in client or public interest; and when cooperative action has client approval.

Fees and Expenses

12. Whether singularly or in joint venture the professional fee, whenever possible, should be determined and explained to the client in advance recognizing such considerations as the nature and scope of the service to be rendered; time required; the consultant's ability, experience and reputation; responsibility assumed by the consultant as well as the benefits which will accrue to the client.

13. The AAHC member shall offer no rebates or other form of recognition to a member of the client family, to an architect, or to any other outside influential person or body in effort to obtain a commission.

14. The consultant shall accept no payment or payments in kind, directly or indirectly, from contractors, equipment manufacturers, or suppliers in recognition of any recommendations or approval he/she makes or gives.

15. The consultant should make every effort to conserve and/or minimize expenditures of the client regardless of the affect on his/her professional fee.

Publicity and Solicitation

16. Promotional activities, paid or other, by member consultants or their firms shall be acceptable when aimed at improving public understanding of the art and science, practice and role of health services consultants and/or the dignified presentation of qualifications to prospective clients and otherwise consistent with all of the preceeding and following herein.

17. The AAHC Consultant shall not advertise firm or personal consultant services in self-laudatory language or in an exaggerated, misleading or false manner.

18. Under no circumstances shall the AAHC logo be used by any individual or firm; however, an individual may use on his/her own letterhead or firm stationery in relationship to his/her name thereon, the name of the Association and his/her membership classification.

19. Identification of individual consultants as members of the American Association of Hospital Consultants is encouraged as in the

by-line of a contributed article to a magazine, in an editorial footnote, or in the descriptive title of a speaker or delegate.

Grievance Procedure

20. To be considered by the Association a complaint or charge against a member must be filed in writing with the Ethics Committee. The Ethics Committee has responsibility for reviewing all written charges and complaints filed and shall promptly acknowledge and investigate such charges on the basis of AAHC Bylaws and this Code of Professional Ethics.

21. The AAHC staff is under obligation to provide the accused member with a copy of the complaint and the opportunity to respond.

22. The respondent will subsequently be provided with a copy of the Committee's findings and recommendations whereupon he/she will be provided a reasonable opportunity for appeal. Such appeal will be heard by the Executive Committee and its decision shall be final.

(Revised August 15, 1975)

Reprinted with the permission of the American Association of Hospital Consultants

Once a selection is made, the consulting process will usually require a great deal of interaction between the consultant and key employees throughout the organization. The quality of information received by the consultant could, in large measure, depend on his respectful acceptance by these key people in the organization. Therefore, to receive maximum benefits from the consultation, top management should try to create an organizational climate that will tap the creative energies of employees throughout the organization and encourage from them the cooperation required.

The professional consultant is governed by a code of ethics, which establishes standards for the practice of his profession. The chief characteristics of the professional consultant are integrity, objectivity, analytical skill, specialized knowledge, broad experience, and a practical approach to the solution of problems. Health institutions should carefully select consultants for these attributes and then expect them to carry out the assignment in accordance with the highest standards of the profession. In turn, the consultant should expect that top management has prepared the organization and has created a climate that attempts to develop positive attitudes and perspectives to make planning and implementation possible.

Notes

1. Max S. Wortman and Leland I. Forest, "Monitoring Consulting Activities—A Revealing Analysis," *Academy of Management Proceedings* (August 19-22, 1973): 172-178.
2. Association of Consulting Management Engineers; American Association of Hospital Consultants.
3. The "Code of Professional Ethics" and "Obligations of Good Practice" appear in *Professional Practices in Management Consulting* (U.S.: Association of Consulting Management Engineers, Inc., 1966), pp. 93-99.

Suggested References

American Hospital Association. "Statement on the Selection of a Consultant for Hospitals and Related Health Care Institutions." in *The Process of Planning in Health Care Institutions*. Chicago: American Hospital Association, 1973. pp. 89-94.

Flath, Carl I. "The Health Facilities Consultant: Qualities He Needs for Efficacy." *Hospital Topics* 48 (March 1970): 33, 36-38.

Flath, Carl I. "How the Consultant Works." *Hospital Topics* 48 (April 1970): 40, 44-46, 99.

Professional Practices in Management Consulting. U.S.: Association of Consulting Management Engineers, Inc., 1966.

Wortman, Max S. and Forst, Leland, I. "Monitoring Consulting Activities—A Revealing Analysis." *Academy of Management Proceedings*. (August 1973): 19-22.

Chapter 8

Outline of a Hospital Long Range Plan

Although long range planning today is crucial to institutional survival, most health institutions will implement a planning process such as described in this book for the purpose of creating a written long range plan of development to be used in conjunction with receiving new program approval from external planning bodies. The existence of such a plan will normally be required to justify major capital expenditures under state certificate of need programs. Presented in this chapter as Exhibit 8.1 is a suggested table of contents for a long range planning study with descriptions of what those contents would entail. Though the plan suggested should be basic to the needs of most health care institutions, individual situations might dictate additions or deletions to fit unique circumstances.

I. INTRODUCTION

Purpose of this Plan:
The primary purpose of the long range plan, which in this case is to define the future role of the institution and develop a long range plan for fulfilling this role.

Approach to the Study:
Describes the rationale for the way in which the plan was developed, including its major components and how the components fit together. For example, the development of this plan was approached in six phases:

1. development of a planning process,
2. analysis of the community served and its resources,

3. development of mission and role,

4. identification of future programs and services **and** their utilization,

5. evaluation of the facility, and

6. development of a plan of implementation.

Exhibit 8.1

TABLE OF CONTENTS
of
A HOSPITAL LONG RANGE PLAN

II. THE PLANNING PROCESS

Planning Philosophy:
States the basic institutional philosophy that guided the development of this plan. For example, this institution sought to develop new programs and services only after a thorough study of the community and its needs and potential relationships with other institutions. Further, the process was designed to include the impact of key individuals both inside and outside the institution.

Planning Participants:
The role of the governing body, administration, and particularly the medical staff and community should be clearly delineated as this is an important aspect of project review by planning bodies. A statement of how individual participants were selected and the methods by which their deliberations were structured would also be of value, not only giving proper acknowledgments but also understanding how the final product was derived.

Endorsements:
Provides evidence of the plan's endorsement by the board, medical staff, and key community institutions and groups. Often, letters of endorsement are attached.

III. THE COMMUNITY SERVED

Service Area:
Presents the methodologies used to identify the population groups served by the institution and describes the geographic, political, natural, or other boundaries that encompass those areas.

Service Area Charxcteristics:
Describes the characteristics of the population residing within the institution's service area with projections of future changes in population growth and composition. Considers future changes in the character of these communities including governmental planning and services, industrial and business

development, and other factors that can affect the need for future health services.

IV. COMMUNITY HEALTH NEEDS AND RESOURCES

Forecast of Community Needs:
Presents the methodologies used to forecast the future health program needs of the areas served, considering population and community changes and the expected utilization of health services by that population. Reviews the guidelines and pronouncements of external planning bodies and either confirms or suggests revisions to forecasted area health needs.

Existing Resources and Services:
Describes the nature and scope of the area's health institutions and the services they provide to the study population. Examines the availability of physician and other health manpower.

Service Gaps or Duplications:
Compares forecasted community needs with the provision of existing services to identify present and future gaps or excesses. Describes health services not now provided by community health resources and examines service competition or program and facility duplications.

V. MISSION AND ROLE OF THE INSTITUTION

Mission Statement:
States the reason for the institution's existence and its overall purpose in the community's health care delivery system.

Roles and Relationships:
Describes the part the institution plays along with other health institutions in the community and its present or planned cooperative relationships in the provision of health services to the area's population.

VI. PROGRAMS AND SERVICES

Historical Utilization:
Describes the existing programs and services of this institution and traces their historical utilization by the population served. Identifies, where possible, the internal or external factors responsible for past utilization patterns.

Planned Programs and Services:
Based on the stated mission and role, and considering the identified gaps and duplications in community health services, this section describes the institution's short and long range plans to carry out service programs in inpatient care, ambulatory care, diagnostic and treatment services, education, research and others that might be relevant.

Projected Utilization:
Projects future utilization of the institution's planned programs and services. Provides statistical information for future program, manpower, facility, or financial planning.

VIII. FACILITY EVALUATION

Physical Facilities:
Presents a description and an evaluation of existing physical facilities and their capacity to respond to the needs of planned programs and services.

Manpower:
Examines the institutional manpower complement and its capacity to respond to planned programs and services. Provides a detailed analysis of medical staff composition and their support of the institution through patient admissions and referrals.

Operations and Finxnces:
Analyzes the operating statistics of the institution with particular emphasis on financial position and capacity to incur further debt.

VIII. IMPLEMENTATION PLAN

Program Priorities:

Places planned programs and services into short and long range priorities and establishes a phased plan for their implementation. Discusses the factors affecting these decisions on priorities and describes the planning assumptions that should be periodically reexamined as each phase of the plan is implemented.

Physical Facility Requirements:

Delineates the requirements for facility modernization, expansion, contraction, or relocation that might be necessitated by each phase of the program plan.

Manpower Requirements:

Describes the numbers and types of manpower needed to staff future programs. Delineates what recruitment efforts or other manpower planning will be required as each phase of the plan is implemented.

Financial Requirements:

Delineates the additional financial resources needed to implement each phase of the plan, with particular emphasis on estimated capital expenditures.

Chapter 9

A Review of the Past and a View to the Future

The history of hospital planning in the United States has been filled with trial and error. Voluntary planning in the early 60s introduced the health industry to the notion that areawide planning was in the best interest of the community. Most areawide planning agencies were organized around a concern for hospital beds, but they relied primarily on voluntary compliance by health institutions. Areawide planning agencies had very little influence over institutional decisions to expand or add new programs unless federal grants or subsidies were involved. Decision making by these agencies was to a great extent influenced by hospital administrators who, in most cases, were given the opportunity to direct the decision making process through their advisory committees. Hospital expansion, duplication, and cost escalation continued unabated, and the handwriting was on the wall: if planning was going to succeed health institutions needed new incentives and planning agencies needed more clout.

When Comprehensive Health Planning Agencies (CHPs) were established under P.L. 89-749, a second generation of hospital planning was ushered in. Created under a broad new federal law these CHP agencies were to be designed to overcome many of the shortcomings of the voluntary planning agencies. First, CHPs had a legal basis for their existence and had government financing. Second, domination of community planning decisions by providers was to some extent mitigated by the requirement that CHP boards have a consumer majority. Third, the scope of planning agency concerns was broadened beyond the focus on hospital beds to include a "comprehensive" view of health care problems and programs.

Yet CHPs were unable to effectively influence hospital planning decisions. There were few instruments at their disposal by which they could request other than voluntary compliance by health institutions. While CHP boards had consumer majorities, decisions were in most cases influenced by the persistence of knowledgeable, hardworking concerned providers who had a vested interest in leading the process. One of the serious problems that inhibited the ability of CHPs to reach their potential was that it took many of them so long to become organized because of the requirements placed upon them by the law. The requirements for representation, the committee structure and assignments, the process of selection and appointment, and the organization and policy development necessary, all delayed the implementation of improved planning methodologies in health institutions.

In spite of these shortcomings, however, CHPs became more sophisticated in the review and comment process, and health institutions had greater community pressure to become more sophisticated in their planning. But CHPs still felt they had little clout to make their recommendations stick, and promoted a debate on certificate of need laws in an increasing number of state legislatures. The outcome of these efforts was that by the early 1970s no more than a couple of dozen states had passed stiff new planning laws. With the continued acceleration of health care costs, Congress already disturbed over the unexpected cost overruns of the Medicare program, began to explore new federal initiatives to control future costs. Under P.L. 92-603, Section 1122 of the Social Security Act was amended to require a certificate of public need when a major captial expenditure by a health institution would result in expected reimbursement for patient care under federal reimbursement programs. Institutions that rejected federal reimbursement programs could still plan outside of the purview of those state agencies administering the 1122 law, and they did. It would appear that 1122 was only a stopgap measure to control Medicare costs until a more comprehensive national health planning law could be passed by Congress.

Health institutions face a new challenge under the National Health Planning Resources and Development Act. The challenge is to improve hospital planning in this country, not by following the dictates of those who may plan by default, but by providing the models and the leadership to make sound planning succeed. "Planning by default" will be carried out by Health Systems Agency (HSA) planners as they attempt to implement the "letter of the law," when health institutions passively wait for planning direction. Planning inaction by health institutions will therefore constitute an open invitation for more centrally directed planning by public bodies.

To carry out the "planning law" HSA staffs will face many of the same problems that plagued their predecessors, the CHPAs. First, planning methodologies in the health field are still somewhat rudimentary, with few receiving wide professional acceptance in practice. Second, few health agency planners have a firsthand understanding of the problems and complexities of planning development and implementation in a health institution. Third, few health planners are really adequately trained for the jobs they will be asked to carry out.

But some form of planning will be implemented, in spite of our present capabilities. Those who will take the time and effort to make hospital planning happen will have a law to help them implement whatever they find necessary. Passive resistance to planning on the part of health institutions will therefore lead to active direction by others. But such does not have to be the case.

The nation has a virtually untapped resource of expertise in management planning. As a prime function of every manager of a health institution, planning is carried out daily to resolve issues and implement programs. But, such planning while expertly carried out by most hospital executives has been short range in nature. Long range planning just focuses on different issues and requires different information for decision making. The process of planning development and implementation, however, utilizes the same management techniques as short range planning.

Hospital executives are therefore in a unique position to help community planning executives design and implement sound planning systems. If they take the initiative, they can lead the community planning process rather than be led. If they can demonstrate the success of planning models and approaches within their own institutions and service areas, planning agencies will be the first to adopt and promote these demonstrations. If they enthusiastically involve the community and get their support for planning efforts, planning agencies will be quick to recognize the merit of these plans.

Health institution executives cannot permit planning to fail. If they lose the initiative, or attempt to block the process, then hospital planning will probably fall short of public expectations. If the public is not satisfied, and if planning is allowed to fail, then the history of U.S. industry would suggest that hospital planning will be centrally regulated and controlled from Washington. However, I believe that health care executives will meet the challenge for reasons related to the changing nature of hospital incentives.

Historically, there have been few positive incentives for long range planning by a health institution. Liberal cost reimbursement by third party payors removed the incentive for accurate demand forecasts and sound fiscal management. An examination of costs versus benefits for major capital expenditures was infrequently employed, with philanthropy often supplying the excess funds required for poorly conceived programs. Benefit patterns of health insurance reduced an institution's flexibility to plan for inadequately reimbursed services, like ambulatory care or outpatient diagnostic services. Graduate schools of hospital administration did not give much attention to the health care manager's long range planning function and consequently the health industry has been deprived of managers who possess these important skills.

But the nature of the industry and the profession of hospital administration is rapidly changing. Increasing regulations and controls over reimbursement and the entire management function are making it almost impossible to continue planning "by the seat of the pants." Patterns of financing capital expenditures have changed with more institutions entering the bond markets and incurring long term debt and fewer relying on philanthropy and government grants. Debt financing has placed new planning requirements on the health care executive.

In the future, capital expenditures by hospitals will be tied to financially feasible programs as lending bodies, whether public or private, will expect sound business decisions based on defensible plans. More accurate hospital planning will be needed to assure fiscal solvency, and many over extended institutions will go bankrupt, as competition for revenue sources increases. More accurate patient demand projections will be required, since arbitrarily raising patient rates to balance the budget will disappear as a tool of modern hospital management. Hospital rates will be under close public scrutiny as will most other aspects of hospital operations. Community, not for profit hospitals will truly become community hospitals with full public disclosure and greater participation by community residents in hospital planning.

Future hospital executives will, therefore, have numerous positive incentives for long range planning. First, the most favorable financing terms and highest bond ratings will go to those institutions with a good track record of sound planning. Second, fiscal solvency will require accurate revenue forecasts as sources for subsidizing financially weak institutions become increasingly scarce. Third, greater public disclosure and community involvement will necessitate long range planning which is truly responsive to population expectations if long term community good will and support is desired. In the future, health institutions will be measured by how well they carry out their pronounced goals and by the effectiveness of their financial management.

Some institutions will attempt to beat the system. They will develop nicely sounding goals, objectives and plans, and go through all of the motions necessary to gain planning agency approval. They will take advantage of the lack of planning sophistication in some communities. In this setting, planning will be guided by the philosophy that the end (i.e., getting a certificate of need) justifies any means necessary for that attainment. Unfortunately, some institutions will get away with this kind of planning with the true victim being the community and its residents, when unneeded and duplicated facilities or service continue to increase hospital costs. Further, poorly utilized facilities will not provide a sufficient volume of patients in those specialities and services for which lack of activity reduces staff competence and therefore quality of care. But, patients will continue to become more discriminating users of hospitals and physicians. Public disclosure and greater community involvement will make it increasingly difficult for a hospital to operate for other than the best interest of the community.

A number of hospitals will develop well thought out long range plans which run contrary to the guidelines of their local Health Systems Agencies. Since community health planning is not yet very precise, and available techniques are only as good as the judgment of the individuals who employ them, health systems agencies will face some challenges. Planners for individual hospitals will have a vested interest to employ a level of expertise which may effectively challenge the assumptions or methods of community planners. Some of these challenges will end up in the courts, the outcomes of which will set precedents for future planning. But this competition will improve hospital planning. In efforts to survive in the face of increasing regulation and control, hospitals will seek the best planning advice available to help them advocate their positions. This competition for the most informed planning input will improve the state of the art.

Like always, politics will play an important role in community planning decisions. Although the boards of Health Systems Agencies will be composed of consumer majorities, experience with Comprehensive Health Planning Agencies suggests that providers will really dominate the decision making process, by virtue of their strong vested interest, special knowledge, and unbroken involvement. But good politics without good planning will ultimately fail. The real test of planning success will be outcomes measured in terms of adequate long term financing, accurate revenue projections, community support and improved community health. In the future, poor planning will threaten the long term survival of a health institution, as it should. Hospitals will no longer be immune from uncertainties of the marketplace and the strategic planning requirements that are a fact of life in the management of American industry.

Index

147

About the Author

Martin S. Perlin is the Director of Health Services for the Central Region of Cresap, McCormick and Paget Inc. He received his B.S. degree from Emory University and both an M.B.A. and a D.B.A. degree from The George Washington University. Dr. Perlin has served in administrative and planning positions in major community hospitals, and has directed a number of long range planning studies for health institutions. At McKeesport Hospital, McKeesport, Pennsylvania, he served as an Assistant Director with responsibility for coordinating a major expansion program and developing an institutional planning process. He held the position of Assistant to the Executive Vice President at the Albert Einstein Medical Center, Philadelphia, Pennsylvania, where he also served an administrative residency in hospital administration. Prior to joining Cresap, McCormick and Paget, Dr. Perlin held a faculty position at the Department of Hospital and Health Administration, Medical College of Virginia. In that position he was responsible for health institution planning, hospital design and construction, community research and health economics. He was also the department's Director of the Community Research Program.

For his doctoral dissertation Dr. Perlin conducted a "Nationwide Survey of Long Range Planning in the Hospital Industry." His research involvement has also included the position of Research Associate on a Public Health Service research grant awarded to the Sisters of Mercy of the Union. He also served as a principal investigator under a grant from HEW in a study of the feasibility of developing and implementing a coordinated system of health care delivery on the eastern shore of Virginia.

Currently, Dr. Perlin is counseling health institutions on the development and implementation of long range plans, program development, facility planning and design, capital financing and certificate of need approval.